Real Stories of

NURSING
RESEARCH

The Quest for
Magnet Recognition

Edited by:

M. Maureen Kirkpatrick McLaughlin, PhD, RN
Georgetown University Hospital
Washington, DC

Sally A. Bulla, PhD, RN
Wake Forest University Baptist Medical Center
Winston-Salem, North Carolina

JONES AND BARTLETT PUBLISHERS
Sudbury, Massachusetts
BOSTON   TORONTO   LONDON   SINGAPORE

World Headquarters

Jones and Bartlett Publishers
40 Tall Pine Drive
Sudbury, MA 01776
978-443-5000
info@jbpub.com
www.jbpub.com

Jones and Bartlett Publishers
Canada
6339 Ormindale Way
Mississauga, Ontario L5V 1J2
Canada

Jones and Bartlett Publishers
International
Barb House, Barb Mews
London W6 7PA
United Kingdom

Jones and Bartlett's books and products are available through most bookstores and online booksellers. To
contact Jones and Bartlett Publishers directly, call 800-832-0034, fax 978-443-8000, or visit our website
www.jbpub.com.

Substantial discounts on bulk quantities of Jones and Bartlett's publications are available to corporations,
professional associations, and other qualified organizations. For details and specific discount information,
contact the special sales department at Jones and Bartlett via the above contact information or send an
email to specialsales@jbpub.com.

The authors, editor, and publisher have made every effort to provide accurate information. However, they are
not responsible for errors, omissions, or for any outcomes related to the use of the contents of this book and
take no responsibility for the use of the products and procedures described. Treatments and side effects
described in this book may not be applicable to all people; likewise, some people may require a dose or
experience a side effect that is not described herein. Drugs and medical devices are discussed that may have
limited availability controlled by the Food and Drug Administration (FDA) for use only in a research study or
clinical trial. Research, clinical practice, and government regulations often change the accepted standard in this
field. When consideration is being given to use of any drug in the clinical setting, the health care provider or
reader is responsible for determining FDA status of the drug, reading the package insert, and reviewing
prescribing information for the most up-to-date recommendations on dose, precautions, and contraindications,
and determining the appropriate usage for the product. This is especially important in the case of drugs that are
new or seldom used.

Production Credits

Publisher: Kevin Sullivan
Acquisitions Editor: Emily Ekle
Acquisitions Editor: Amy Sibley
Associate Editor: Patricia Donnelly
Editorial Assistant: Rachel Shuster
Associate Production Editor: Katie Spiegel
Marketing Manager: Rebecca Wasley

V.P., Manufacturing and Inventory
  Control: Therese Connell
Composition: Cape Cod Compositors, Inc.
Cover Design: Timothy Dziewit
Cover Image: © Ann Trilling/ShutterStock, Inc.
Printing and Binding: Malloy, Inc.
Cover Printing: Malloy, Inc.

Library of Congress Cataloging-in-Publication Data
Real stories of nursing research : the quest for Magnet recognition / [edited by] M. Maureen McLaughlin and
    Sally A. Bulla.
        p. ; cm.
    Includes bibliographical references and index.
    ISBN 978-0-7637-6166-0
    1. Nursing—Research.   I. McLaughlin, M. Maureen.   II. Bulla, Sally A.
    [DNLM: 1. American Nurses Credentialing Center. Magnet Recognition Program.   2. Nursing Research.
3. Awards and Prizes.   4. Nursing Service, Hospital—standards.   WY 20.5 R2877 2010]
RT81.5.R428 2010
610.73072—dc22

                                                                                    2009001854
6048

Printed in the United States of America
13 12 11 10 09   10 9 8 7 6 5 4 3 2 1

In memory of my parents, Joseph E. and Sarah C. Kirkpatrick,
who made multiple sacrifices so their children
could get a better education.
M. M. K. M.

In honor of my family for their continued support over the years.
S. A. B.

Contents

Informatics

Intensive Care

PART VII: ADDITIONAL RESOURCES

Foreword

Nursing historian Eleanor Lambertsen (1958) summarized the history of nursing from the pioneering period of the late 1800s, through periods of standards-setting in the early 1900s, to the 1950s, when the nursing profession determined its societal relevancy through data collection. From that time forward, Morrison (1960) suggested that the contributions of nurses would "bend the course of the future" (p. 75). Now, 50 years later, the future is now, and the Magnet Recognition Program has indeed bent the course of modern nursing.

The 15-year history of the Magnet program is familiar to all of us. The program has its roots in a pivotal 1983 study by McClure, Poulin, Slovie, and Wandelt that identified 14 critical factors in a hospital environment that would attract and retain qualified nurses. According to the American Nurses Credentialing Center (ANCC; http://www.nursecredentialing.org), 41 of the 163 institutions in the 1983 study were described as "magnet" hospitals because they had the ability to attract and retain highly qualified professional nurses. In 1990, the then-Magnet Hospital Recognition Program for Excellence in Nursing Services was created, and in 1994, the University of Washington Medical Center in Seattle became the first ANCC-designated Magnet organization. Since that time, hundreds of American healthcare organizations have successfully achieved Magnet status. This coveted designation revolves around the well-known "Forces of Magnetism" associated with excellence in nursing, recognizes quality patient care and innovations in professional nursing practice, and provides consumers with a practical benchmark for selecting the hospitals where they can expect good care. In addition to credentialing, the Magnet program plays an important role in disseminating best practices in nursing.

Since 1990, a large literature has evolved on the organizational characteristics, best practices, quality indicators, leadership requirements, and outcome data associated with the Magnet program. Now, Drs. M. Maureen Kirkpatrick McLaughlin and Sally A. Bulla have compiled this wonderful book of nursing

stories—*Real Stories of Nursing Research: The Quest for Magnet Recognition*—
that allows us to share in the real life experiences of American nurses who have
sought the Magnet designation. The title of this sets the stage for some fascinating learning. The title first tells us that we can expect to enter the world of these
21st century nurses not through endless tables of statistical data but through the
power of their own words, their own stories, and their own experiences. The title
also tells us that the challenging journey of these nurses is similar to heroes in
mythology (from the Greek word *mythos*, which means *story*) and the literature
of the past.

The use of real nursing "stories" about the Magnet experience is a communication approach that is as old as humankind but relatively new in nursing. As
Sawyer said in 1942, and as Campbell and Moyers reminded us in 1988, the history,
poetry, and laws of the past have been kept alive and passed from generation to
generation by the oral tradition. In 1993, Neuhauser suggested that storytelling is
the single most powerful form of human communication—a method for inspiring,
teaching, comforting, and entertaining—and the primary tool that human beings
use to pass on their cultures. Neuhauser has said that in today's organizations,
stories—in the form of legends of the past and what she called "sacred bundles"—
help to create employee buy-in and the desire to support the legends or become
even better legends themselves. Such stories also reflect the changing nature of
organizational cultures via changes in organizational structure, products, strategy, and/or technology. In the business world, for example, Shaw, Brown, and
Bromiley (1998) said that "stories are a habit of mind at 3M, and it's through them—
through the way they make us see ourselves and our business operations in complex, multi-dimensional forms—that we're able to discover opportunities for
strategic change. Stories give us ways to form ideas about winning" (p. 42).

Neuhauser (1993) and Boyce (1996) have told us that stories are powerful
tools to use in the type of work that involves team building, building mission and
vision, and influencing employee morale and customer satisfaction. Shaw et al.
(1998) added that "storytelling and planning are related . . . a good story and a
good strategic plan define relationships, a sequence of events, cause and effect
and priority among items—and those elements are likely to be remembered as
a complex whole. That argues strongly for strategic planning through storytelling" (p. 42). Brown and Duguid (2000) concluded very simply that "storytelling helps us discover something new about the world and allows us to pass
that discovery to others" (p. 6). Thus, in their focus on storytelling in nursing, Drs.
McLaughlin and Bulla have used an ancient technique to give voice to the work
of many nurses and nursing teams, to the planning of strategy, to the changing
culture of healthcare organizations and, most important, to the discovery of
what is possible in and for the nursing profession of today.

The voices of nurses in this book are presented not in isolation but in the context of a hero's adventure or quest that is undertaken under adverse and challenging circumstances. We know from folklore, mythology, and literature that a quest is a journey in which a hero or adventurer leaves the comfort of home to seek a very important goal that can benefit the greater good. Barrette's 1999 analysis of the structure of quests gives us some insights into what readers can expect from this enlightening nursing text. Barrette details the ways in which the hero accepts the challenges of the quest: The hero reaches out to companions to accompany her along the long journey, receives help, exerts great effort, faces many obstacles, considers suspending the quest, enters another world quite different from where she came, overcomes fears, and, ultimately, beats the odds to triumph by obtaining the cherished object of the quest.

As you read *Real Stories of Nursing Research: The Quest for Magnet Recognition*, you will be walking with the courageous nurses who left their comfort zone in a quest for one of nursing's greatest rewards: the Magnet designation. Enjoy their stories, and enjoy the journey.

Joyce E. Johnson, PhD, RN, NEA-BC, FAAN
CNO and Senior VP of Operations
Georgetown University Hospital
Washington, DC

REFERENCES

Barrette, P. (1999). *The quest in classical literature: Structuralism and databases.* Retrieved December 10, 2008, from http://www.iath.virginia.edu/ach-allc.99/proceedings/barrette.html
Boyce, M. E. (1996). Organizational story and storytelling: A critical review. *Journal of Organizational Change Management, 9*(5), 5–26.
Brown, J. S., & Duguid, P. (2000). Balancing act: Capturing knowledge without killing it. *Harvard Business Review, 78*(3), 73–80.
Campbell, J. (with Moyers, B.). (1988). *The power of myth.* New York: Doubleday.
Lambertsen, E. C. (1958). *Education for nursing leadership.* Philadelphia: J. B. Lippincott Co.
McClure, M., Poulin, M., Slovie, M., & Wandelt, M. (1983). *Magnet hospitals: Attraction and retention of professional nurses.* Kansas City, MO: American Academy of Nursing.
Morrison, L. J. (1960). *Steppingstones to Professional Nursing.* St. Louis: Mosby.
Neuhauser, P. C. (1993). *Corporate legends & lore: The power of storytelling as a management tool.* New York: McGraw-Hill.
Sawyer, R. (1942). *The way of the storyteller.* New York: Compass Books.
Shaw, G., Brown, R., & Bromiley, P. (1998). Strategic stories: How 3M is rewriting business planning. *Harvard Business Review, 76*(3), 3–8.

Preface

This book evolved from a study we did in 2006 for which we asked the question, "How do nurse researchers at Magnet hospitals implement nursing research programs?" Researchers from 112 Magnet hospitals reported that there was a lot of nursing research being conducted at their hospitals. However, they also reported the inability to disseminate the findings of these studies because of rejections of their proposals for publication and presentations. We took that as an opportunity to help share the research studies being done by clinical nurses and to get the abstracts from those nursing studies published. Although we received calls and messages from several doctorally-prepared nurses who wanted to be contributors for this book, we graciously (we hope) declined their offer. We informed them that our strategic intention was to include only stories from nondoctoral nurses to demonstrate their successes with research. Our intention is that perhaps nurses who read these stories and abstracts will be inspired by our contributors' stories and also overcome that fear of research. (You can do it!)

How did we get nurses to contribute their stories and abstracts for this book? The strategy we used to obtain these stories was to distribute approximately 2,000 "call for stories" flyers at the 2007 American Nurses Credentialing Center Magnet Conference in Denver, Colorado. This outreach strategy resulted in contributions from more than 70 nondoctoral nurses from 14 U.S. states and the District of Columbia who work in small and large hospitals located in rural, urban, and suburban areas.

The purpose of this book is to demonstrate how non-doctoral-prepared nurses in clinical settings overcame their fears of research and went on to conduct nursing research studies. This information is conveyed in individual or team stories, along with an abstract from a research study that these nurses conducted.

This book is divided into seven parts. Part I, Overcoming the Fears of Research, consists of two chapters authored by nurse researchers who address how to overcome the fear of research and the importance of research as it relates to Magnet designation.

Part II, Resources Novice Researchers Can't Do Without, has four chapters, one each by a nurse researcher, a statistician, a medical outreach librarian, and a nurse representative from an institutional review board (IRB). These chapters focus on the importance of individual collaboration with a mentor, a librarian, and a statistician, and provide tips for submitting your proposal to the IRB.

Part III, Research Stories Related to Evidence-Based Practice (EBP), consists of eight chapters written by nondoctoral nurses who tell stories of EBP and how it relates to their research journey.

Part IV, Research Stories Related to Medical-Surgical Nursing Areas, comprises 12 chapters that reflect a variety of stories and studies done by medical-surgical nurses.

Part V, Research Stories Related to Nursing Specialty Areas, consists of 37 chapters representing studies from the specialties of emergency services, end-of-life care, informatics, intensive care, maternal and child health, neonatal intensive care, oncology, orthopedics, pediatrics, and post-anesthesia care unit.

Part VI, Research Stories Related to Education, Development, and Retention Issues, consists of five chapters and addresses some of the most important issues of research as they relate to assisting bedside nurses through continued education and development.

Part VII, Additional Resources, comprises a glossary, frequently asked questions (FAQs), a list of online nursing research resources, and three views on the future of nursing research from industry leaders.

It is our hope that if you learn one thing from this book, it is this: If all the nurses in this book can do nursing research, *you* can do nursing research too!

Our very best wishes,

M. M. K. M. and S. A. B.

Acknowledgments

A very special thank you to Emily Ekle of Jones and Bartlett who listened to our idea for this book, believed it had the potential to inspire other nurses to seek research opportunities, and encouraged us to send her our manuscript. We would also like to acknowledge Rachel Shuster and Katie Spiegel of Jones and Bartlett for the kind and gentle manner in which they provided ongoing assistance throughout the production process. In addition, the authors gratefully acknowledge the following:

To all the contributors for their stories and abstracts that they enthusiastically sent to us in order to help inspire other nurses to overcome their fear of research, we thank you! A special thanks to Elaine Scherer, Dr. Nawar Shara, Ivonne Martinez, and Kim Groner for their contributions as experts in their respective topics.

To Dr. Joyce E. Johnson for writing the foreword and for hiring me to get "nurses excited about research" at Georgetown University Hospital (GUH) in Washington, DC. (In addition to getting GUH nurses excited about research, I discovered a new exciting phase of my nursing career that I enjoy tremendously!) A big dose of gratitude goes to Dr. Molly Billingsley for her encouragement and support of all of our research endeavors. Also, thanks to Judy Poller for her assistance in compiling and organizing information for us. And to our families for their ongoing love and support, always.

M. M. K. M. and S. A. B.

Contributors

Steven T. Anderson, BSN, RN
Rex Healthcare
Raleigh, NC

Laurel Barbour, RN, APN
Advocate Lutheran General Hospital
Park Ridge, IL

Sylvia M. Belizario, BSN, MEd, CNRN
MedStar Health/Georgetown University Hospital
Washington, DC

Butch O. Blake, ADN, RN
Barnes-Jewish Hospital
St. Louis, MO

Diane Braun, BSN, MA, CCRP
Advocate Christ Medical Center
Oak Lawn, IL

Janet Brock, ADN, RN
University of Virginia Health System
Charlottesville, VA

Megan E. Brunson, BSN, RN, CCRN-CSC
Saint Joseph's Hospital of Atlanta
Atlanta, GA

Barb Bungard, BSN, RN, CCRN
Akron Children's Hospital
Akron, OH

Judith Cavanaugh, MSN, RN-BC
Advocate Christ Medical Center
Oak Lawn, IL

Denise Cedeno, BS, RN
Our Lady of Lourdes Memorial Hospital
Binghamton, NY

Alison Chappell, BSN, RN, CMSRN
MedStar Health/Georgetown University Hospital
Washington, DC

Suzanne S. Clark, RN, ACHRN
Morristown Memorial Hospital
Morristown, NJ

Maria Coussens, RNC
University of California, Irvine Medical Center
Orange, CA

Cathleen M. Daley, MS, RN
St. Peter's Health Care Services
Albany, NY

Tina Daniels, RN, RNC
Pinnacle Health Neonatal Intensive Care
Harrisburg, PA

Patricia Conway Decina, BSN, RN, CPN
Bryn Mawr Hospital/Pediatric Unit of the Main Line Health System
Bryn Mawr, PA

Cynthia Earley, BSN, RN
Inova Loudoun Hospital
Leesburg, VA

Linda Eaton, MN, RN, AOCN
Oncology Nursing Society
Pittsburgh, PA

Kathleen Fitzgerald, MSN, RN, ACM
Winchester Hospital
Winchester, MA

Susan Fowler, PhD, RN, CNRN, FAHA
American Association of Neuroscience Nurses
Glenview, IL

Mary Ann Francisco, MSN, CCRN, CNS-BC
University of Chicago Medical Center
Chicago, IL

Donna Grochow, MS, RNC
University of California, Irvine Medical Center
Orange, CA

Kimberly H. Groner, MSN, RN, CANP, CCRC
MedStar Health/Georgetown University Hospital
Washington, DC

Jane H. Hartman, MSN, RN, CPNP
Cleveland Clinic
Cleveland, OH

Jocelyn D. Holmes, MS, RN
University of Chicago Medical Center
Chicago, IL

Renee Houser, LPN, Lead Clinic Nurse
Penn State Milton S. Hershey Medical Center
Hershey, PA

Irene Huntzinger, RN, CNOR
Upper Valley Medical Center
Troy, OH

Nancy B. Hutchison, MS, RN, CCRN
Saint Joseph's Hospital of Atlanta
Atlanta, GA

Audrey Jones, MSN, RN
Riverside Methodist Hospital
Columbus, OH

Lou Ann Jones, MSN, APRN, BC
Inova Heart and Vascular Institute
Leesburg, VA

Julie A. Kenney, BSN, RNC, CMSN
Advocate Christ Medical Center
Oak Lawn, IL

Sharon Kimball, MS, RN, CNL, CRRN
Providence Acute Rehabilitation Center
Portland, OR

Carol Korman, MSN, RN, BC
Akron Children's Hospital
Akron, OH

Ruth M. Labardee, BSN, RNC
Riverside Methodist Hospital
Columbus, OH

Phyllis Lawlor-Klean, MS, RNC, APN/CNS
Advocate Christ Medical Center/Hope Children's Hospital
Oak Lawn, IL

Mary Beth Leaton, MS, RN, CCRN, APN
Morristown Memorial Hospital
Morristown, NJ

Christina Lloyd, MS, RNC
Children's National Medical Center
Washington, DC

Paula Lomas, BSN, RN, CCRP
Morristown Memorial Hospital
Morristown, NJ

Stephanie A. Lopuszynski, BSN, BS, RN
Saint Joseph's Hospital in Atlanta
Atlanta, GA

Peggy Malone, BS, RN, OCN, OSF
OSF St. Anthony Center for Cancer Care
Rockford, IL

Sandra Marconi, RN,C
Penn State Milton S. Hershey Medical Center
Hershey, PA

Ivonne Martinez, MLIS
Georgetown University
Washington, DC

Jean M. Mau, BS, MSN, RN, APN
Advocate Lutheran General Hospital
Park Ridge, IL

Amy Hall McCowan, MEd, RN, CMSRN
Penn State Milton S. Hershey Medical Center
Hershey, PA

Dena McCoy, BSN, RN
Children's National Medical Center
Washington, DC

Elizabeth Miller, BSN, RN
Children's National Medical Center
Washington, DC

Deborah Morehouse, MSN, RN
Children's National Medical Center
Washington, DC

Tamara H. Murphy, MS, ACNS-BC, CCRN
Penn State Milton S. Hershey Medical Center
Hershey, PA

Katherine Nagy, MS, APRN, BC
St. Peter's Hospital
Albany, NY

Cheryl G. Newmark, BSN, RN
Morristown Memorial Hospital
Morristown, NJ

Sherry (Sharon) Ninni, BSN, RN, CCRN
Morristown Memorial Hospital
Morristown, NJ

Mildred O'Meara-Lett, BS, RN, CCRN
Inova Loudoun Hospital
Leesburg, VA

Sheree O'Neil, MSN, RN
Inova Loudoun Hospital
Leesburg, VA

Caryn Peters, RNC, RRT
Morristown Memorial Hospital
Morristown, NJ

Gwen B. Phillips, BSN, RNC
Riverside Methodist Hospital
Columbus, OH

Wendy Ploegstra, MSN, RN, CCRN
The University of Chicago Medical Center
Chicago, IL

Susan E. Powers, MS, RN
Winchester Hospital
Woburn, MA

Gail Probst, MS, RN, CNA, ANP, OCN, AOCN, BC
Huntington Hospital
Huntington, NY

Laura Reilly, MSN, CCRN, CNRN
Morristown Memorial Hospital
Morristown, NJ

Jeanne M. Rorke, MSN, RNC, NNP
MedStar Health/Georgetown University Hospital
Washington, DC

Sally Rudy, MSN, RN
Penn State Milton S. Hershey Medical Center
Hershey, PA

Elaine M. Scherer, BSN, MA, RN
Magnet Recognition Program
Mountain Area Health Education Center
Asheville, NC

Nawar M. Shara, PhD
MedStar Research Institute
Hyattsville, MD

Sue Stott
Academy of Medical-Surgical Nurses
Pitman, NJ

Mary Beth Strauss, MS, RN, BC
Winchester Hospital
Winchester, MA

Carol Swartz, RN
Lourdes Center For Family Health DePaul Pediatrics
Binghamton, NY

Brigitte Taylor, RNC
Inova Loudoun Hospital
Leesburg, VA

Shelley Thibeau, MSN, RNC
Ochsner Medical Center
New Orleans, LA

Catherine Tieva, BA, RN, OCN
St. Cloud Hospital
St. Cloud, MN

Sharon Truitt, RN, CCRN
Pinnacle Health System
Harrisburg, PA

Lisa Waraksa, BS, RN, CPN
Bryn Mawr Hospital
Bryn Mawr, PA

Cindy Ward, MS, RNC, CMSRN
Centra Health, Lynchburg General Hospital
Lynchburg, VA

Laura Waszak, RN
Advocate Christ Medical Center/Hope Children's Hospital
Oak Lawn, IL

Rosanna Welling, MBA, RN
Advocate Christ Medical Center/Hope Children's Hospital
Oak Lawn, IL

Lisa Williams, BSN, RN
Children's National Medical Center
Washington, DC

Amy E. Winecoff, BSN, RN, COHN-S
Lake Norman Regional Medical Center
Mooresville, NC

CHAPTER 1

What's So Scary About Nursing Research?

M. Maureen Kirkpatrick McLaughlin

If you ever told me I'd be writing a chapter for a book about overcoming fears of nursing research, I'd say you were over the edge and beyond saving! I only became involved with research because it was a requirement for me to complete my doctoral program. Research is something I never would have considered if I didn't have to, so I understand the hesitancy and fears of nurses as they relate to taking the research path. But as I tell nurses all the time, "If I can do nursing research, *you* can do nursing research!"

Now, several years later, I find myself getting excited (I know, I can hardly believe I'm saying that!) about the opportunities for nursing research. I feel like our profession is only at the very tip of a very deep iceberg as it relates to nursing research, and we have a lot of exploring to do beneath the surface. I hope that like me, you too (if you haven't already) will take the plunge and learn how rewarding conducting research can be.

WHAT IS SO SCARY AND INTIMIDATING ABOUT NURSING RESEARCH?

It's that unknown factor. The idea, pervading our thinking, that "we can't do research." Not true! Many nurses may not be aware of the role that each of us is expected to fill in pursuing research, nor the resources that are available to help us make it happen. Years ago, nursing research was not part of the standard nursing curriculum, and nurses were perceived by many as "handmaidens"—certainly not research professionals who asked, and solved, the *why* and *what if* questions related to problems associated with health care. Back then, conducting nursing research was not an expectation of the nurse who provided clinical care at the bedside, but today it is. So, for many of the approximately three million nurses out there today who were not educated or trained in research methods, it can be very scary and intimidating. Of course, please be reassured that once that fear is faced, like other fears, it is overcome.

1

Many nurses lack an interest in research, feel that they are "too old to learn new tricks," or are intimidated by data that require statistical analysis. I know that the thought of having to "do statistics" scared me to death—until I took a statistics course. (And yes, the only reason I took it was that it was required!) As my former statistics professor told me, "You aren't taking this course to become a statistician, but to learn how statistics is applied in health care. When you need to do statistics, consult with a statistician, they are the experts in that field." Those words gave me a deep sense of relief because statistics is "not my thing." It gave me permission (so to speak) to focus my attention on other areas of research and allowed me to not be intimidated by statistics. For those nurses who are not comfortable with statistics, I highly recommend establishing a collaborative, consultative relationship with a statistician. Statisticians are an important part of your research team; you will learn a lot from them as you work together and discuss your research study, and they will help you to overcome the fear and intimidation factor.

Unlike nurses trained in the past, many student nurses today are exposed to the importance of nursing research. Many nursing programs mandate statistics and research courses that help students learn about the importance of research within nursing. The tricky thing is to have these novice nurses continue on with research activities—such as implementing the research proposal they had to do in school—in their clinical setting. Want to be a research scientist? One hospital, Lehigh Valley Hospital in Allentown, Pennsylvania, is teaching nurses to be "bedside scientists" (Houser & Bokovoy, 2007).

MYTHS AND FEARS

Nurses come up with all sorts of justifications as to why they can't or shouldn't do research. Do any of the following excuses sound familiar?

- It's not my job. (Oh yes it is!)
- I have to have an advanced degree. (No you don't.)
- I have to do statistics. (No you don't.).
- I don't have the skills. (You can learn them!)
- I don't have anyone to help me. (Find someone.)
- I don't understand research terminology. (Learn it.)
- I'm not a good writer. (Get help from someone who is!)
- I don't have time. (Make it.)
- I don't have the money to do the study. (Seek funding.)
- I don't have the support of my manager. (Keep after them!)

These are nothing but excuses because each of them can be overcome. Talk to any nurse who had some of these same fears and addressed them head-on. He or she will tell you it can be done! All nurses need to do is to take the outstretched hand of other nurses (and nonnurse resources) willing to help them. Repeat after me: "If *you* can do nursing research, I can do nursing research!"

WHY DO NURSES NEED TO OVERCOME THESE FEARS?

There is a new expectation of the clinical nurse, especially in Magnet-designated hospitals. And with the increased number of hospitals seeking Magnet status, many hospitals are challenged to integrate research within their own settings. This is because at least seven specific criteria related to evidence-based practice (EBP) and research (addressed in Force 6: Quality of Care in the Magnet documentation) are sought as evidence by the 2005 American Nurses Credentialing Center's (ANCC) Magnet Recognition Program®:

1. Describe how current literature appropriate to the practice setting is available, disseminated, and used to change administrative and clinical practices.
2. Discuss the institution's policies and procedures that protect the rights of participants in research protocol. Include evidence of consistent nursing involvement in the governing body responsible for protection of human subjects in research.
3. Provide evidence that research consultants are actively involved in shaping nursing research infrastructure, capacity, and mentorship.
4. Provide a copy of the nursing budget or other resources of funding for the past year, the current year-to-date, and the future projection, highlighting the allocation and utilization of resources for nursing research.
5. Supply documentation of all nursing research activities that are ongoing, including internal validation studies, internal and external research, and participation in surveys completed within the past 12-month period.
6. Provide evidence of education and mentoring activities that have effectively engaged staff nurses in research and/or evidence-based practice activities.
7. Describe resources available to nursing staff to support participation in nursing research and nursing research utilization activities. (American Nurses Association, 2005, p. 4)

However, the new model for ANCC's Magnet Recognition Program®, which has been restructured and is similar to a report card, will present outcomes addressed by Force 6 criteria in Section V, Empirical Quality Results (American Nurses Credentialing Center).

Nurses are expected to be part of an interdisciplinary research team that will help improve health care by translating research into practice and demonstrating positive outcomes. In addition, clinical nurses are expected to conduct research that will not only apply to patient care, patient safety, and patient quality but also encompass a broader reach, to include nursing practice and the workplace environment.

Regardless of how many nurses think that research "is not my job" because of their education level, it has an important role for them to play. According to LoBiondo-Wood and Haber (2006), there is agreement that individuals at all levels of professional nursing, from the nurse with an associate's degree to the nurse with a doctoral degree, have a need for research skills. Some examples of these skills follow.

Associate Level

- Demonstrates awareness of the relevance of research to nursing
- Helps identify problem areas in nursing practice
- Assists in data collection activities
- Uses research findings in practice appropriately
- Participates as team members

Baccalaureate Level

- Understands each step of the research process
- Generates clinical questions that require investigation
- Participates on research teams
- Collects and records data
- Shares research findings with colleagues

Master's Level

- Is an active member of a research team
- Provides clinical expertise and evidence-based knowledge
- Serves as a champion for change
- Provides leadership
- Conducts research as a coinvestigator or investigator

Doctoral Level

- Appraises, designs, and conducts research
- Develops theoretical explanations of phenomena
- Develops studies using quantitative and qualitative methods
- Serves as a role model and mentor to guide other nurses

- Collaborates/consults with other agencies on research endeavors
- Disseminates research findings to scientific community via journals, conferences, etc. (LoBiondo-Wood & Haber, 2006, pp. 9–11)

Nurses who are not already familiar with the research process will hear and learn more about it as hospitals continue to hire doctoral-prepared nurses to implement nursing research programs. In a national study done by McLaughlin, Billingsley, and Bulla (2007), nurse researchers at 112 Magnet hospitals identified strategies and facilitators that they used to implement their nursing research programs, as well as barriers. The top three strategies identified by these nurse researchers for implementing nursing research programs within their hospitals were (1) having an active role with the hospital's nursing research council, (2) being members of nursing research study teams at their hospitals, and (3) using formal nursing research protocols. In addition, these nurse researchers reported that their professional activities in assisting nurses with research included (from highest to lowest frequency) mentoring other nurses, developing research questions, assisting with literature reviews, reviewing and editing proposals, completing institutional review board (IRB) paperwork, and analyzing findings. Respondents from this study reported that research activities, such as journal clubs and research education sessions, were being provided on-site at these hospitals (McLaughlin, Billingsley, & Bulla, 2007).

To make these education programs more appealing, many hospitals also provide compensation for participating nurses, such as paying their hourly wage to attend these classes. Another plus for nurses who attend these sessions is obtaining continuing education contact hours and a certificate of attendance for their professional portfolios.

Although most research classes are designed to accommodate a group of nurses, as opposed to a nursing research internship/fellowship program that may provide 1:1 information, education, and mentoring by a nurse researcher, both are very effective. Both of these outreach methods can make a difference in reducing the level of fear a nurse may have about research. In fact, these methods help to increase the knowledge and the confidence that nurses can learn an additional new skill, conducting research, just like they have learned all their other skills, from basic to advanced. But can it be fun?

FUN HELPS FIGHT FEARS

Providing research education in a nonthreatening and fun way can help to fight the fear of research. For instance, two fun research seminars presented to nurses at Georgetown University Hospital were "A Recipe for Research" and "CSI and EBP." The Recipe for Research seminar made a comparison between following a recipe for a luscious dessert and a recipe for a research study. Visual aids for this presentation included a cook's hat, an apron, "the recipe," pots and pans, mixing bowls, and spoons and other utensils. At the end of the presentation, participants were asked to write out on a "recipe card" one ingredient (action step) that they would use to promote nursing research on their unit. Even if nurses don't like to cook, they can still understand the process!

Another fun education session highlighted the popular TV program *CSI–Las Vegas* to demonstrate and compare crime scene investigation (CSI) with clinical science investigation. Music, a toolkit, and "Who always wanted to be an actor/actress?" engaged the nurses. The music from *CSI* ("Who Are You?") was played at the beginning and throughout the presentation to set the stage and get participants into a relaxed frame of mind. "Investigative tools" were extracted from a "CSI Toolkit" and discussed by the investigators (nurses who volunteered to play the roles of the television CSI characters Grissom and Katherine). Comparisons were made of the tools used for crime scene investigations and tools used for clinical science investigations, and the importance of following an investigative protocol. Awards for participation were provided to the "actors and actresses." Research doesn't have to be boring, a major complaint from many nurses who don't want to pursue it. Research can be educational and fun! "Edutainment" can be a powerful tool to engage nurses about research and help them overcome their fears. And use your resources!

USE YOUR RESOURCES

How do nurses get started in nursing research? (see **Table 1-1**). Nurses need to remember to use any and all resources they can to help them with their research. This includes librarians, statisticians, and nurse representative reviewers from the IRB. See other chapters in this book for words of wisdom from these experts!

LINK THEORY TO PRACTICE

Novice researcher one day, expert researcher of the future! It is inspirational to watch clinical nurses overcome their fear of research and make the

Table 1-1   Ten Easy Steps to Get Involved in Research

1. Start simple. Identify other nurses interested in research. Think about questions that arise from your practice that could be explored.
2. Start reading research articles related to a topic that interests you.
3. Form a unit or hospital-based journal club to discuss research articles.
4. Identify others conducting research in your hospital and join their team.
5. Contact a colleague at another hospital and join their research team.
6. Identify what research topics your nursing specialty is addressing. (Check their Web site.)
7. Identify a research study that can be easily replicated on your unit.
8. Identify a nursing research mentor (nurse researcher, college professor).
9. Identify internal resources to help you (librarians, ethicists, researchers).
10. Identify external resources to help you (colleges of nursing, national nursing specialty organizations, Sigma Theta Tau, etc.).

Source: McLaughlin, M. M. (2007). Overcoming fears of nursing research. *Advance for Nurses, 9*(20), 29.

connection between theory and practice. I have seen them identify a problem on their unit; conduct a literature review to find out what others have done (or not) to address the problem; formulate a hypothesis/research question based on their search of the literature; identify a population, sample type, and size; develop a research design; create their own measurement tools; and establish face and content validity of a specific instrument through networking with national experts. I have seen nurses learn how to design data collection forms, assign codes to data for statistical analysis (to be applied by the statistician), and share their research results via poster and podium presentations at national presentations. You can too!

How do nurses overcome their fear? Read on further in this book and see for yourself! And remember, if I can do nursing research, *you* can do nursing research!

REFERENCES

American Nurses Association. (2005). *Magnet Recognition Program application manual 2005.* Washington, DC: Author.

American Nurses Credentialing Center. (2008). *Announcing a new model for ANCC's Magnet Recognition Program.* Magnet Recognition Program. Retrieved November 19, 2008, from http://www.nursecredentialing.org/Magnet/NewMagnetModel.aspx

Houser, J., & Bokovoy, J. (2007). *Clinical research in practice: A guide for the bedside scientist.* Sudbury, MA: Jones and Bartlett.

LoBiondo-Wood, G., & Haber, J. (2006). *Nursing research: Methods and critical appraisal for evidence-based practice.* St. Louis, MO: Mosby-Elsevier.

McLaughlin, M. M., Billingsley, M., & Bulla, S. (2007). *Implementation of nursing research programs in Magnet Hospitals in the U.S.* Unpublished manuscript, Georgetown University Hospital, Washington, DC.

CHAPTER 2

What Does "Magnet" Have to Do with Research?

Sally A. Bulla and Elaine M. Scherer

THE MAGNET PROGRAM: A HISTORY LESSON

Magnet actually got its start as a research question. In 1981, the American Academy of Nursing (AAN) appointed the Task Force on Nursing Practice in Hospitals. Its purpose was to conduct a study to identify and describe variables that created an environment that attracted and retained well-qualified nurses who promoted quality patient, resident, and client care. Of the 155 hospitals originally contacted, 46 were deemed Magnet for purposes of the study, but only 41 participated. These original 41 institutions are referred to as magnet hospitals because of their ability to attract and retain professional nurses. According to Maggie McClure, the chair of the original task force and a researcher on the team, it was radical at that time to look at why nurses stayed at certain facilities (McClure, Poulin, Sovie, & Wandelt, 1983). The Chief Nursing Officer and the staff nurses in these 41 reputational hospitals were interviewed to identify the characteristics that seemed to distinguish these magnet organizations. These characteristics became known as the "Forces of Magnetism" (American Nurses Credentialing Center, 2008a).

The Magnet Recognition Program® was developed by the American Nurses Credentialing Center (ANCC) to recognize healthcare organizations that provide nursing excellence. The program recognizes quality patient care and innovations in professional nursing practice and serves as a vehicle to disseminate these successful nursing practices and strategies. The Magnet Recognition Program® also provides consumers with the ultimate benchmark to measure the quality of care they can expect to receive (American Nurses Credentialing Center, 2008a).

In 1990, the American Nurses Association board of directors approved the initial proposal for the Magnet Hospital Recognition Program for Excellence in Nursing Service. Following a pilot program that included five facilities, the University of Washington Medical Center in Seattle became the first ANCC-designated Magnet organization. The program has continued to change and expand through the years and now includes more than 300 facilities, including long-term care facilities and hospital organizations abroad (American Nurses Credentialing Center, 2008a).

MAGNET AND THE RESEARCH CONNECTION: A DISCUSSION WITH ELAINE M. SCHERER, FORMER DIRECTOR OF THE MAGNET RECOGNITION PROGRAM®

Research is the key to advancing the science of nursing and the nursing profession, so it was natural for research to eventually become an integral piece of the "Forces of Magnetism." Although a part of the "Forces of Magnetism" almost from the inception of the program, before 2003–2004, formal research programs in healthcare facilities were limited. Once research was highlighted in the 2005 Magnet manual, it became an integral part of the recognition program.

As hospitals and nursing services have progressed on their Magnet journey, nurses have become more comfortable participating in research studies. The nursing profession understands and respects the direct impact that the knowledge gleaned from nursing research studies has on the improvement of care. As more nurses participated in research studies, they began to lead studies, coming up with their own researchable questions about their nursing practice.

Initially, the scoring components of development, dissemination, and enculturation were key elements in the evolution of research. These elements clearly described the importance of having Magnet standards become part of the culture rather than a policy sitting on the shelf. The research component has, however, led to some confusion. Facilities, early in their Magnet journey, have often confused quality improvement initiatives, evidence-based practice initiatives, and research. As the emphasis on research grew, nurses and facilities began to identify the *so what?* question that is integral to research. By asking the *so what?* question, nurses began to see how research could be used to highlight the improvement in patient outcomes.

THE MAGNET APPRAISER AND RESEARCH: THE DISCUSSION CONTINUES

One oft-asked question is: What do the Magnet appraisers look for regarding the research component? There is not a check-off list. The appraisers are looking for a culture that is rich in research. Research has to be part of the culture. In general, the appraisers find it easy to determine whether research is just a term, or whether it is actively lived in the organization; is it part of the enculturation process in the organization?

The Chief Nursing Officer sets the tone for the entire facility by his or her leadership. It becomes evident when research is valued by the Chief Nursing Officer and the facility. Once nurses begin doing research, it becomes more than just a line item in a budget; research becomes a living standard of practice throughout the organization. In smaller facilities that have fewer resources, there was a tremendous amount of creativity seen in partnerships and in the use of part-time researchers from other organizations.

There are other key components that appraisers can identify in organizations with cultures rich in research. One key component is that all types of education are encouraged and supported at all levels. A second component is that the Chief Nursing Officer is experienced and comfortable with research. An organization with a rich culture in research will have at least one PhD on staff, or a creative partnership with another facility or university to share research resources.

Another key to a culture rich in research is mature nursing staff. These mature staff have mastered their nursing duties and are able to branch out into the research process. Facilities with a majority of newer nurses have a different culture, one in which the nurses are trying to learn their basic nursing skills and figure out what specialty area is right for them. Many may not be ready to include research in their daily nursing routines unless they had positive experiences in their nursing research courses and conducted studies to meet course requirements.

The appraisers look carefully at facilities that have a significant focus on the medical model. These facilities have nurses who may be involved in research studies and who are comfortable getting involved in research as part of their nursing duties; however, they may or may not be involved in nursing research. Facilities that have an active nurse representative on their institutional review board also are more involved in nursing research.

Last but not least, many successful facilities make research a part of their practice by discussing it with new nurses as they start at the facility. This is often done by integrating evidence-based practice and research into orientation programs, preceptor programs, and internships. Many hospitals are now also discussing research at interviews with applicants as part of job expectations.

THE NEW MODEL

The ANCC has announced a new model for the Magnet Recognition Program®. This new model was developed to provide more clarity and direction and combines the 14 Forces of Magnetism into five model components. This approach was designed to put greater focus on measuring outcomes, to streamline documentation, and to eliminate redundancy. The goal of this new model is to showcase how Magnet organizations have made a difference.

These outcomes will be addressed in terms of clinical outcomes related to nursing, workforce outcomes, patient and consumer outcomes, and organizational outcomes. Through these outcomes, a Magnet-recognized organization will have a simple way of demonstrating excellence (American Nurses Credentialing Center, 2008b).

In addition to the new model, the ANCC is endeavoring to establish a national research agenda for the Magnet organizations. The ANCC conducted its first National Magnet Research Agenda study from October 2005 to February 2006. Seventy-nine organizations participated in this study. Nurse researchers and executives were surveyed. The ANCC plans to conduct periodic surveys to continue to develop the most important research priorities for healthcare organizations (American Nurses Credentialing Center, 2008c).

Twenty-six research topics judged to have the highest priority by both researchers and executives were developed as a result of the survey. These research topics were combined into five categories: clinical outcomes, patient and nurse satisfaction, organizational/practice environment, human resources, and financial and material resources (American Nurses Credentialing Center, 2008c).

The clinical outcomes were divided into five topics: quality of care, errors, adverse events, injuries, and functional outcomes. The patient and nurse satisfaction category consisted of patient satisfaction with the overall nursing care, patient satisfaction with pain management, RN satisfaction with his or her current job, RN satisfaction with physician–nurse relationships, and RN satisfaction with management/administration (American Nurses Credentialing Center, 2008c).

The organization/practice environment category had five main topics: evidence-based practice, effective leaders, quality improvement processes, staff relationships, and failure to rescue. The human resources category consisted of seven topics: adequacy of nurse staffing, RN retention, RN education levels, advanced practice nurses as knowledge resources, RN vacancy rates, RN certification levels, and support service staff. The final category is financial and material resources, which consists of four main topics: cost savings due to improved patient safety, cost savings due to RN retention, professional development opportunities, and funds for professional development (American Nurses Credentialing Center, 2008c).

The advancement of nursing science is vital to the profession of nursing. Research will continue to be a key component of the Magnet Recognition Program®. It is vital for nurses at Magnet facilities and facilities that aim to achieve Magnet status to continue their pursuit of nursing excellence by identifying nursing issues, embarking on the research process to answer these issues, and continuing the quest for quality patient care.

REFERENCES

American Nurses Credentialing Center. (2008a). *Program overview*. Magnet Recognition Program. Retrieved November 19, 2008, from http://www.nursecredentialing.org/Magnet/Program Overview.aspx

American Nurses Credentialing Center. (2008b). *Announcing a new model for ANCC's Magnet Recognition Program. Magnet Recognition Program*. Retrieved November 19, 2008, from http://www.nursecredentialing.org/Magnet/NewMagnetModel.aspx

American Nurses Credentialing Center. (2008c). *National Magnet research agenda*. Magnet Recognition Program. Retrieved November 19, 2008, from http://www.nursecredentialing.org/ FunctionalCategory/AboutANCC/CredentialingResearch/NationalMagnetResearchAgenda.aspx

McClure, M. L., Poulin, M. A., Sovie, M. D., & Wandelt, M. A. (1983). *Magnet hospitals: Attraction and retention of professional nurses*. Washington, DC: American Nurses Association.

CHAPTER 3

Nurturers: The Importance of Mentors

M. Maureen Kirkpatrick McLaughlin

Did you know that the most rewarding part of many nurse researchers' jobs is to mentor other nurses? It's true! According to a study by McLaughlin, Billingsley, and Bulla (2007), 71% of nurse researchers at Magnet hospitals self-reported "mentoring other nurses" as one of their top professional activities. In addition, these same nurse researchers reported that mentoring was one of the top three facilitators for implementing their nursing research programs in their hospitals and that for many, it was the "most rewarding part of the job"! See, nurse researchers *are* ready and willing to be your mentor!

One of the best ways to nourish a nurse with research is to provide him or her with a mentor. I wish I'd had a mentor early in my nursing career. I have witnessed the transformation that having a mentor can make in a nurse's self-confidence level. It can help to take a level of confidence "lower than snake spit" to a high mountaintop like Mount Everest.

Many young and inexperienced nurses unfortunately had the unpleasant experience of "being eaten" by older nurse coworkers who thought they were more knowledgeable. How sad and embarrassing that is for our profession. How can we expect our nurses to grow and develop professionally if they aren't "fed" the nourishment they need? Instead of "eating our young," mentors are best known for "feeding our young." They are "gourmets" who provide rich experiences and resources that whet the taste buds of less experienced nurses for just how good a nursing career can be.

WHAT IS A MENTOR?

Definitions of *mentor* may vary, but the bottom line is that a mentor is a person with experience helping another person with less experience. Think in terms of a teacher, coach, counselor, advisor, advocate, or role model. Do you have a mentor? Do you want a mentor? Would you like someone to take a special interest in you both personally and professionally? I often picture a mentor like a guardian angel, lovingly hovering over a person to help guide him or her on a safe (but sometimes rocky and challenging) career path, whispering, "Watch out for that landmine!" or "Be careful, there's a shark!"

MENTOR PROGRAMS

There are different types of mentoring programs, some more formal than others. Most will include a mentor and a mentee (or protégé). According to Byrne and Keefe (2002), there are multiple models, including the traditional mentor and mentee/protégé model, and team and peer models. The best model for you will be the one that fits *you*. There is no "one size fits all" because we all have different personalities and different learning styles. That's why it's very important to find a research mentor whom you will feel comfortable with. You know the type—the mentors who will say, "Ask me anything. There are no stupid questions. If you don't ask, you will never know." You want a mentor who will encourage you to ask questions; you know that he or she will explain the answer to you until you fully understand it, and asking won't make you feel like an idiot!

CHARACTERISTICS OF MENTORS

The characteristics of mentors will vary, but many have the following attributes as they relate to working with a mentee/protégé:

- a desire to see their mentee/protégé succeed
- frequent and easy availability to the mentee/protégé
- excellent communication skills, especially good listening skills
- a positive, helpful, nonintimidating, and caring attitude
- the willingness to share and give resources of interest to the mentee/protégé
- the ability to challenge the thinking of the mentee by helping to stretch his or her brain muscles in a "cerebral gym"
- the ability to be nonjudgmental
- a high level of integrity and trustworthiness
- serve in a role as both teacher and student
- facilitate growth and development experiences
- celebrate success!

FINDING A MENTOR

Are you looking for a research mentor but don't know where to find one? Places where you can find them include hospitals, universities, regional research consortiums or societies, national research organizations, and national nursing specialty organizations. For convenience, you might want to check first within your hospital to see if there is a nurse researcher employed there. Depending on the size of the hospital, this role may be filled with a researcher in a full-time or part-time position, or perhaps someone in a consultant role. If your hospital hasn't hired a nurse researcher yet, you can check with the nursing research faculty at an area university's college or school of nursing.

Research mentors can be found in regional nursing research consortiums. For example, the Washington Regional Nursing Research Consortium in Washington, D.C., comprises multiple clinical and academic nurse researchers from the surrounding metropolitan area, which includes the District of Columbia, Virginia, and Maryland. One of the goals of this consortium is for members to serve as mentors to novice nurse researchers.

E-MENTORING

So you aren't sure about having a mentor at your workplace? No problem. How about an e-mentor? This type of mentor will communicate with you electronically and help guide you from a distance. Have you heard of GEM nursing? It is a Group Electronic Mentoring (GEM) in Nursing program, geared toward a population younger than 21, that promotes nursing as a career and then links high school students with nurses who volunteer to be mentors (Kalisch, Falzetta, & Cooke, 2005).

Perhaps you would prefer a mentor from a distance, yet only a click away. You can always contact a regional nursing research society and see if there is a mentor there who meets your needs. Examples of regional nursing research societies are the Eastern Nursing Research Society (http://www.enrs-go.org), the Midwestern Nursing Research Society (http://www.mnrs.org), the Southern Nursing Research Society (http://www.snrs.org), and the Western Institute of Nursing (http://www.ohsu.edu/son/win).

Nursing specialty organizations may also employ nurse researchers who can provide a mentorship. These mentors can be located by contacting a specific nursing specialty organization. For example, critical care nurses interested in research can contact the American Association of Critical-Care Nurses (http://www.aacn.org), operating room nurses can contact the Association of periOperative Registered Nurses (http://www.aorn.org), and oncology nurses can contact the Oncology Nursing Society (http://www.ons.org) and ask for a research mentor. In addition, part of the mission of the Council for the Advancement of Nursing Science (http://www.nursingscience.org) is to "facilitate life-long learning opportunities for nurse scientists," and this organization has multiple nurse researchers as its members.

ASK AND YOU SHALL RECEIVE

There is a saying that "when the student is ready, the teacher will appear." When a novice researcher is ready to learn, a mentor will somehow show up to provide the learning opportunities that the student seeks. What are these research opportunities? More than you know! A research mentor can introduce you to, and help you to get excited (seriously!) about, discovering answers to questions that can make a significant clinical or statistical difference in nursing. Think of it as taking an exciting TRIP to places yet discovered!

A TRIP YOU WON'T WANT TO MISS

What is it about nursing that interests you? What would you like to learn more about? Your research mentor can brainstorm with you to help you identify a clinical question that you may want to pursue by researching it. Along that trip, the mentor may introduce you to, or refamiliarize you with, research terminology such at PICO, EBP, and the Iowa Model. Most important, he or she will help you learn to translate research into practice (TRIP). Further, your mentor can assist you in developing your research design, advise and review your methodology, connect you with a statistician, assist you with the institutional review board forms, review the research findings with you, and discuss the limitations and implications of research. The research mentor can also help you with grant writing to seek research funding. In addition, he or she can also help you seek opportunities to disseminate your findings at regional and national conferences and get published. The greatest advantage of having your very own research mentor is that he or she can expose you to the entire research process in a nonthreatening environment, one in which you will be nurtured and will thrive (See **Table 3-1**).

Now doesn't that sound like an exciting TRIP you'd like to take?

Table 3-1   Research Mentors

Research mentors can:
M   motivate, model, and move the mentee/protégé forward in research
E   enthuse, engage, educate, and explain research to the mentee/protégé in a safe environment
N   nurture the needs of the novice mentee/protégé through networking with colleagues
T   teach, translate, and provide the time it takes to travel with the mentee/protégé on the research trip
O   open minds and doors with outreach opportunities to help the mentee/protégé discover the thrill of research
R   reflect to reassess the way in which they "role model" research to the mentee/protégé to make it irresistible!

REFERENCES

Byrne, M., & Keefe, M. (2002). Building research competence in nursing through mentorship. *Journal of Nursing Scholarship, 34*(4), 391–396.

Kalisch, B. J., Falzetta, L., & Cooke, J. (2005). Group e-mentoring: A new approach to recruitment into nursing. *Nursing Outlook, 53*(4), 199–205.

McLaughlin, M. M., Billingsley, M., & Bulla, S. (2007). *Implementation of nursing research programs in magnet hospitals in the U.S.* (Unpublished). Georgetown University Hospital, Washington, DC.

CHAPTER 4

Lessons from a Librarian

Ivonne Martinez

As a hospital outreach librarian, it is my ultimate goal to ensure that nurses maximize their ability to access and effectively use current information resources and technology. I hope this brief overview will be a good beginning for all your future research projects.

Often nurses seek the library's services to assist them with their research projects. Services range from instruction on how to use the library's electronic resources for information retrieval, to reference assistance, research consultations, and literature searches. Librarians, also known as information professionals, are trained to provide relevant, current, and accurate information. As a health sciences librarian, I cannot say enough about the work that we do. In today's complex healthcare environment, there is the need for expertise to access the plethora of information sources available.

In most instruction sessions on library resources, I explicitly explain how a librarian can maneuver through all the online resources available. How can I be of assistance to nurses? I can assist nurses from the moment a research idea is conceptualized all the way to manuscript preparation and publishing. For instance, at a recent library instruction session, I taught a group of nurses about library resources and services and, in particular, which of those services/resources would assist nurses in starting their research project. The session consisted of topics such as setting up library accounts, developing a search strategy (see Appendix A), learning research best practices (see Appendix B), searching the literature in databases such as PubMed and CINAHL, learning how to use a Web-based bibliographic management software program like RefWorks, and accessing patient information resources (see Appendix C).

Instruction on a library's resources and services is most helpful when held in a computer classroom within the library. In this environment, nurses have the opportunity to actively participate in constructing a search strategy. Nurses can follow the instructions presented by the librarian during the literature search, ask questions as they arise, and get immediate answers. Either way, users—in this case, nurses—may enhance their learning experience by practicing the skills learned in the presence of the librarian (Finley, Skarl, Cox, & VanderPol, 2005).

Most institutions have an array of databases that nurses may use to search the nursing literature. Some of these databases are:

- CINAHL (Cumulative Index of Nursing & Allied Health Literature)— Provides indexing for 2,938 journals from the fields of nursing and allied health. Offering complete coverage of nursing journals and publications from the National League for Nursing to the American Nurses Association, it covers nursing, biomedicine, health sciences librarianship, alternative/complementary medicine, consumer health, and 17 allied health disciplines.
- National Library of Medicine, PubMed—Provides access to citations from MEDLINE and OLDMEDLINE, some general science and chemistry journals, and life science journals.
- Nursing Consult—Mosby's evidence-based medicine tool brings the leading nursing resources together in one integrated online service to help nurses efficiently find answers to pressing clinical questions.
- HealthStar (Health Services Technology, Administration and Research)— Contains citations to the published literature on health services, technology, administration, and research. Focuses on both the clinical and nonclinical aspects of healthcare delivery, such as evaluation of patient outcomes; effectiveness of procedures, services, and processes; administration and planning of health facilities, services, and manpower; health insurance; health policy; laws and regulation; licensure; and accreditation.
- Cochrane Databases of Systematic Reviews—Includes the full text of the Cochrane Collaboration's regularly updated systematic reviews of the effects of healthcare interventions.
- EMBASE—Index to international pharmacological and biomedical literature from over 6,500 journals from 70 countries.
- National Guidelines Clearinghouse—Comprehensive database of evidence-based clinical practice guidelines and related documents.

This is not an inclusive list of all databases, and it is a good practice guideline to consider other databases when searching the literature. A nurse may wish to begin with CINAHL, but databases such as PubMed, Cochrane Library, or EMBASE may be applicable to nursing. Such highly specialized databases may take some time to learn, but a librarian can offer a mediated search or, if you prefer, meet one on one with you and instruct you on how to use some of these databases.

Instruction of resources and database searching are services that librarians can offer, but there are other important roles that many of us take on. Take, for example, the role of librarians to explore evidence-based nursing. In this role, the librarian conducts and filters systematic searches, obtains articles, and appraises and summarizes results (Tod, Bond, Leonard, Gilsenan, & Palfreyman, 2007).

Another important support service that a librarian provides concerns the validation process for hospitals with Magnet designation. Such services include support of research and its integration into the delivery of nursing care, professional development of nurses, and interdisciplinary collaboration (Rourke, 2007). A further role of the librarian involves working with the institutional review board (IRB) team and serving as the main reference contact for primary investigators, clinical trial investigators, and IRB members (Frumento & Keating, 2007).

The ultimate goal of the hospital outreach librarian is to ensure that nurses maximize their ability to access and effectively use current information resources and technology when they need it, wherever they are. If you need more assistance, seek out your hospital or academic health science librarian; it will be his or her pleasure to assist you.

REFERENCES

Finley, P., Skarl, S., Cox, J., & VanderPol, D. (2005). Enhancing library instruction with peer planning. *Reference Services Review, 33*(1), 112–122.

Frumento, K. S., & Keating, J. (2007). The role of the hospital librarian on an institutional review board. *Journal of Hospital Librarianship, 7*(4), 113–120.

Rourke, D. R. (2007). The hospital library as a "magnet force" for a research and evidence-based nursing culture: A case study of two Magnet hospitals in one health system. *Medical Reference Services Quarterly, 26*(3), 47–54.

Tod, A. M., Bond, B., Leonard, N., Gilsenan, I. J., & Palfreyman, S. (2007). Exploring the contribution of the clinical librarian to facilitating evidence-based nursing. *Journal of Clinical Nursing, 16*(4), 621–629.

CHAPTER 5

Statistical Analysis Is a Healthcare Tool

Nawar M. Shara

Many nurses are afraid of statistics, but, like the stethoscope and microscope, statistics is a tool that boosts our observational powers. Statistics is simply the science of making sense of research data in a way that readers can understand and therefore apply the information. Data collection and statistical analysis are two parts of the same tool. When paired correctly, the results can help us to make objective observations that translate into improved disease prevention and patient care. Conversely, like the stethoscope and microscope, if data and statistics are used incorrectly, a faulty observation can lead to an erroneous conclusion.

The purpose of statistical analysis, whether simple or complex, is to test a hypothesis and permit an investigator to make an objective observation. Some studies aim to describe a characteristic in a population; no comparison is made. Some studies aim to compare characteristics or outcomes in two or more groups. In both types of studies, hypothesis testing allows us to make an objective observation through a systemic collection of data. In the studies in which a comparison is made, hypothesis testing determines if the observation was made by chance or if there is a predictable pattern to the data—that is, if there is statistical significance to the observation.

Quantitative studies, whether they consist of simple or complex data collection and simple or complex statistical analyses, share two characteristics:

1. They are based on the scientific method.
2. They use data that are properly matched to a statistical method appropriate for testing the hypothesis.

Do you remember having to do a science project when you were in middle or high school? See, you were a scientist even before you read this chapter! Even back then, you were already doing research and using a "scientific method" to answer a question. Do you remember the process? You most likely followed this method:

The Scientific Method

1. Make an observation.
2. Ask a question about the observation.
3. Turn the question into a testable hypothesis. This can be simple (*There are more men than women in the building today*) or complex (*Drug A is more effective than Drug B in preventing renal failure*).
4. Plan the study; develop a protocol or scientific process that can be repeated by others (replicated).
5. Perform the study.
6. Analyze the results.
7. Evaluate the hypothesis.
8. Share results and conclusions.

It is essential to the success of every study that the hypothesis, or the research question, be clearly stated before data collection begins. In this way, the researcher can ensure that the correct data are collected to test the hypothesis or answer the research question. An ideal data collection procedure is one that measures or captures the variable of interest in a way that is relevant, credible, accurate, unbiased, and sensitive. No method is perfect, but with a little bit of help from a statistician or experienced researcher, some of the pitfalls can be avoided.

To someone inexperienced in data analysis, it may not be immediately apparent what types of data are needed to test the hypothesis. For this reason, the hypothesis should be communicated to a statistician, or a more experienced researcher if a biostatistician is not available. Clinician-investigators are not expected to be experienced statisticians. However, savvy clinician-investigators will consult a statistician while planning a study if at all possible.

A famous use of statistics for disease prevention is an example from John Snow, the father of epidemiology. There was a cholera epidemic in 1854 in Soho, London. At the time, the mechanism of transmission of cholera was unknown. Dr. Snow collected data on the cholera victims and plotted their locations on a map. This allowed him to observe the distribution of the disease in the community. He noticed that an unusually high number of deaths took place near a water pump on Broad Street. This led to Dr. Snow's hypothesis that the water source contributed to the cholera outbreak. To test his hypothesis, he convinced local authorities to remove the pump's handle. After this was done, the number of cholera deaths was dramatically reduced. He then discovered the source of contamination: a leaky cesspool. Dr. Snow later combined data from several outbreaks and used statistics to show a correlation between contaminated water and cholera 30 years before *Vibrio cholerae* was identified.

John Snow shows us two important elements of good health research: (1) he engaged the scientific method, and (2) he used appropriate analysis of the data. The appropriate analysis is what allowed him to make the important observation of disease distribution in a sample of people.

HOW TO TALK TO STATISTICIANS: USE WORDS THEY UNDERSTAND

It's probably been a while since you last had a statistics or research class. Let's go over some definitions.

Variables: A variable is an attribute of a person or object that varies. Differing types of data are turned into differing types of variables used in statistical analysis. There are three basic types of variables: nominal, ordinal, and continuous.

Nominal variables are based on data such as gender, eye color, ethnicity, and disease status (yes/no). There is a finite number of possibilities for each of these variables.

Ordinal variables are based on data such as number of children in family, number of years of college, and stage of disease (I, II, or III). Like nominal variables, there is a finite number of possibilities for each ordinal variable, but unlike nominal data, ordinal values can be ordered from lowest to highest.

Continuous variables are based on data such as age, systolic blood pressure, and body mass index (BMI). Continuous variables differ from nominal and ordinal variables in that continuous variables have infinite possible values for each variable: between any two ages, there is an unlimited number of possible ages. For analysis, age is usually treated in increments of 1 year. Systolic blood pressure can be used in analysis in increments of 1 mmMg or 10 mmMg.

Dependent and independent variables are used when a comparison is made.

The dependent variable is the characteristic of interest, such as blood pressure. It is often the case that there is one dependent variable per statistical test. The investigator wants to make an observation of blood pressure.

Independent variables are characteristics that may have an effect on the dependent variable, such as age, gender, and BMI. There can be more than one independent variable per statistical test. For instance, an investigator wants to observe the effect of BMI on blood pressure (the dependent variable) when the effects of age and gender on blood pressure are controlled.

Descriptive Statistics: Quantitative data would be chaos without statistics, which allows for summarization, organization, interpretation, and communication of the numeric information.

Frequency Distributions: A frequency distribution is a systematic arrangement of the values in a data set from lowest to highest, with the number of times each value was obtained. This arrangement lets us see the range of the variable, the lowest and highest value, the total number of observations n, what the most common value is, and where the observations are mostly grouped. For example, we might find that in our sample, systolic blood pressure ranges from 80(units) to 210(units); that more women than men have diabetes; and that 50% of the sample was older than 60 years. Frequency distributions are often displayed in either a table or a graph.

Central Tendency: Frequency distributions are used for organizing data, whereas central tendency and variation are used for summarizing the data. Examples of central tendency are mean, median, and mode.

The Mean: The mean is widely used in statistics, and it is certainly the most used measure of central tendency. It is computed by summing all scores and dividing by the number of subjects. Many important statistical procedures, especially significance tests, are based on the mean. However, it does have its disadvantages. The mean is affected by each and every score, so one extreme value can change the mean and, in some cases, distort it so that it becomes a misleading value.

The Median: The median is the midway point in a distribution; 50% of the values are below it, and 50% are above it. The median is the average position in the distribution. It is affected by the number of scores only, and, unlike the mean, it is not affected by the magnitude of each score.

The Mode: The mode is the value with the highest frequency in a distribution. Unlike the mean and the median, there can be more than one mode in a distribution, or none at all.

The Range: The range is simply computed from abstracting the lowest value from the highest value. It is highly unstable, because it depends on only two values. The range is often joined with another measure of variability.

Standard Deviation: The standard deviation (*SD*) is the most commonly used measure of variance. It indicates the average amount of deviation of values from the mean.

Null Hypothesis: When a study hypothesis is developed, a corresponding null hypothesis is also developed. For instance, a hypothesis is, *There is a correlation between cigarette smoking and heart disease.* The null hypothesis is, *Cigarette smoking has no effect on heart disease.*

Power: Adequate power, usually defined as 90% or greater, defines the risk of failing to reject the null hypothesis when it is wrong. A study powered at 90% has a 10% risk that the null hypothesis will not be rejected when it should be. Power is determined by the size of the population or study sample, the statistical method needed to test the hypothesis, and the types of variables needed for analysis. Thus, the power of a test is the test's probability of correctly rejecting the null hypothesis.

Significance Level: The level of significance (α) is the probability of rejecting a true null hypothesis. This value can be controlled by the researcher, and the most common value used is .05 and .01. The minimum value selected for α is usually .05. Selecting .05 as the significance level means that out of 100 samples, the null hypothesis will be rejected only 5 times. We do have a problem, though; by decreasing the risk of type I error, we will increase the risk of type II error instead. However, we can decrease type II error by increasing the sample size.

Hypothesis Testing: The research question leads to the hypothesis. A study should have one primary hypothesis and can have additional secondary hypotheses, but one must keep in mind that one study will not answer all questions. Hypothesis testing provides the researcher with objective criteria for deciding whether hypotheses are supported by empirical evidence. However, hypothesis testing is only one piece of evidence that influences the researcher's decision.

Type I and Type II Errors: Statistical inferences are based on incomplete information; therefore, there is always a risk of error. Researchers decide whether to accept or reject a null hypothesis by determining how probable it is that observed group differences are due to chance.

Table 5-1   Type I and Type II Errors

	The null hypothesis is true	The null hypothesis is false
We accept the null hypothesis	Correct	Type II error
We reject the null hypothesis	Type I error	Correct

As the title suggests, there are two types of errors in statistical inference: type I error, which is committed when we reject a true hypothesis, and type II error, which is committed when we accept a false hypothesis.

Statistical Significance: Each of these types of data can be used in comparisons of characteristics. When a comparison is made, determining if the resulting observation was made by chance or if the pattern is predictable, if it is *statistically significant*, is often dependent on the *power* of the study. Results of statistical significance tests are often expressed as the p value.

P value, or probability value, refers to the probability that the data correspond to a predictable pattern or that they appear merely by chance. A p value is commonly considered significant if it is 5% (0.05) or less. This means that there is a 5% (or less) risk that the results were produced by chance. In study results with a p value < 0.05, the research hypothesis (what the researcher is trying to prove) is accepted, and the risk that the null hypothesis (hypothesis of no difference or no effect) is erroneously rejected is 5% or less.

There is much that a researcher needs to know about statistics. Our intent is not to teach statistics but to jog your memory of past classes that you may have had in statistics or research. Nursing research is not done in a vacuum. Gathering a team that includes a biostatistician or an experienced researcher to help you with your research can go a long way in assisting you with your research design, data collection, and analysis. Don't be afraid of research and statistics; get help. There are many people willing to assist you in your research endeavors.

CHAPTER 6

Tips for Completing an IRB Application

Kimberly H. Groner

Congratulations! You've now completed your written proposal. And, it is hoped, you've received news of funding. You are now ready to contact your local institutional review board (IRB) for review of your proposal so that you can conduct this interesting research project.

WHY APPLY TO THE IRB?

Let's begin by discussing why it is that we apply to the IRB or IRC (institutional review committee) prior to conducting any research.

An IRB is established within an institution to assure the safety of research participants. Title 21, Chapter 1 of the Code of Federal Regulations defines IRB guidelines in the United States (46 FR 8975, Jan. 27, 1981). An IRB is any board, committee, or other group formally designated by an institution to review, to approve the initiation of, and to conduct periodic review of, biomedical or behavioral research involving human subjects. The primary purpose of such review is to assure the protection of the rights and welfare of the human subjects (section 520(g)) (46 FR 8975, Jan. 27, 1981).

The membership of an IRB is also outlined in these regulations. Section 56.107 states that IRB membership:

> shall have at least five members, with varying backgrounds to promote complete and adequate review of research activities commonly conducted by the institution. The IRB shall be sufficiently qualified through the experience and expertise of its members, and the diversity of the members including consideration of race, gender, cultural backgrounds and sensitivity to such issues as community attitudes, to promote respect for its advice and counsel in safeguarding the rights and welfare of human subjects. The IRB shall be able to ascertain the acceptability of proposed research in terms of institutional commitments and

regulations, applicable law and standards or professional conduct and practice (U.S. Department of Health and Human Services, 1998).

It is also recommended that an IRB not be composed entirely of men or women and include at least one member whose primary concerns are scientific. In addition, the IRB shall have another member who is not otherwise affiliated with the institution nor part of the immediate family of another IRB member. Individuals with competency in special areas may be invited at any time to review a proposal that requires expertise beyond current members' knowledge.

When an IRB reviews a project, a number of criteria must be met for the project to receive IRB approval:

1. The risks to subjects are minimized as much as possible.
2. The risks to subjects are reasonable in relation to anticipated benefits.
3. The informed consent is adequate.
4. Where appropriate, the research plan makes provisions for the safety of the subjects during the data collection process.
5. Where appropriate, there are adequate provisions to protect the privacy of subjects and maintain confidentiality of data.
6. Appropriate safeguards are included within the study to protect the rights and welfare of the vulnerable subjects.

HISTORICAL OVERVIEW OF HUMAN SUBJECT PROTECTION

In addition, human subject research must conform to the basic ethical principles that govern research involving human subjects. The following section summarizes important events in the development of protections for human subjects in research.

a. *The Nuremberg Code.* The modern history of human subject protections begins with the discovery, after World War II, of numerous atrocities committed by Nazi doctors in war-related research experiments. The Nuremberg Military Tribunal developed 10 principles, known as *The Nuremberg Code*, to judge the Nazi doctors. The significance of the code is that it addressed the necessity to *require the voluntary consent* of the human subject and that any individual "who initiates, directs, or engages in the experiment" must bear personal responsibility for the quality of consent.

b. *The Declaration of Helsinki.* Similar principles have been articulated and expanded in later codes, such as the World Medical Association

> *Declaration of Helsinki: Recommendations Guiding Medical Doctors in Biomedical Research Involving Human Subjects* (1964, revised 1975, 1983, 1989, 1996, and 2000), which calls for prior approval and ongoing monitoring of research by independent ethical review committees.

c. *The Belmont Report.* Revelations about the 40-year United States Public Health Service Syphilis Study at Tuskegee and other ethically questionable research resulted in legislation in 1974 that called for regulations to protect human subjects and for the creation of the National Commission for the Protection of Human Subjects of Biomedical and Behavioral Research to examine ethical issues related to human subject research. The commission's final and most influential report, *The Belmont Report: Ethical Principles and Guidelines for the Protection of Human Subjects of Research*, defines the ethical principles and guidelines for the protection of human subjects. Perhaps the most important contribution of the *Belmont Report* is its explanation of three basic ethical principles: (1) respect for persons (reason for obtaining informed consent); (2) beneficence (explaining and weighing risks and benefits); and (3) justice (fairly selecting subjects). The *Belmont Report* also provides important guidance regarding the boundaries between biomedical research and the practice of medicine (U.S. Department of Health and Human Services, 1979).

REGULATIONS RELATED TO PROTECTING HUMAN SUBJECTS

In addition, the Department of Health and Human Services (DHHS) 45 CFR Part 46, Subpart A, outlines the protection of human subjects. This protection of human subjects is called the Common Rule. These DHHS regulations also include additional protections for pregnant women, human fetuses, and neonates (Subpart B); prisoners (Subpart C); and children (Subpart D). All human subject research must comply with all four subparts of the DHHS regulations. These regulations are enforced by the DHHS Office for Human Research Protections (OHRP) (U.S. Department of Health and Human Services, 1999).

The Food and Drug Administration (FDA) has its own set of regulations. The FDA has also defined *informed consent* (21 CFR Part 50), *IRB regulations* (21 CFR Part 56), and *child protection* (61 FR 20589 and 21 CFR Part 50, Subpart D). These regulations are almost identical to the DHHS regulations.

Additional FDA regulations relevant to the protection of human subjects address Investigational New Drug Applications (21 CFR Part 312), Biological

Products (21 CFR Part 600), and Investigational Device Exemptions (21 CFR Part 812).

In general, FDA human subject regulations apply to clinical investigations and other research involving products regulated by the FDA, including food and color additives, drugs for human use, medical devices for human use, biological products for human use, and electronic products. IRB review and approval is required for clinical investigations and other research involving products regulated by FDA for human use even if an Investigational New Drug Application (IND) or Investigational Device Exemption (IDE) is not required. Simply put, an IRB application must be completed with your institution and the IND or IDE that is filed with the FDA.

Finally, IRBs operate under a Federal Wide Multiple Project Assurance (MPA) or the Federal Wide Assurance (FWA) from the OHRP in the Department of Health and Human Services (DHHS). These policies and procedures apply to all research that involves human subjects, regardless of the source of funding, if any (45 CFR 46.103). It is the responsibility of the institution to assure federal agencies in writing that it will comply with regulations governing the protection of human subjects. As part of this assurance, the institution must develop policies and procedures for conducting human subject research in a responsible and ethical fashion, including how research will be reviewed by the IRB, the reporting of unanticipated problems to the IRB and appropriate regulatory bodies, and other issues.

So, we have reviewed the ethical principles of research and the federal regulations that govern IRBs, and we have listed many of the agencies that define safety in research. Now let's review the types of human subject research.

Federal regulations (45CFR 46.102(d)) define research as "a systematic investigation, including research development, testing, and evaluation, designed to develop or contribute to generalizable knowledge." This is why most IRB applications ask us to explain why and how our research is generalizable to the population at large. This also explains why we must include individuals of varying ages and ethnicities. Federal regulations (45 CFR 46.102(f)) define a human subject as "a living individual about whom an investigator (whether professional or student) conducting research obtains (1) data through intervention or interaction with the individual or (2) identifiable private information." Private information includes information that an individual can reasonably expect will not be made public, and information about behavior that an individual can reasonably expect will not be observed or recorded. Identifiable means that the identity of the individual is known or may readily be discovered by the investigator, or it is associated with the information.

TYPES OF HUMAN SUBJECT RESEARCH

The following examples illustrate common types of human subject research. These are examples only and do not constitute an exhaustive list.

1. *Biomedical research.* Biomedical research involves research to increase scientific understanding about normal or abnormal physiology, disease states, or development, and to evaluate the safety, effectiveness, or usefulness of a medical product, procedure, or intervention. Vaccine trials, medical device research, and cancer research are all types of biomedical research.
2. *Social and behavioral research.* The goal of social and behavioral research is similar to that of biomedical research—to establish a body of knowledge and to evaluate interventions—but the content and procedures often differ. Social and behavioral research that involves human subjects focuses on individual and group behavior, mental processes, or social constructs. It usually generates data by means of surveys, interviews, observations, studies of existing records, and experimental designs that involve exposure to some type of stimulus or environmental intervention.
3. *Clinical research.* Clinical research involves the evaluation of biomedical or behavioral interventions related to disease processes or normal physiological functioning.
4. *Epidemiology research.* Epidemiology research targets specific health outcomes, interventions, or disease states and attempts to reach conclusions about cost-effectiveness, efficacy, interventions, or delivery of services to affected populations. Some epidemiology research is conducted through surveillance, monitoring, and reporting programs—such as those employed by the Centers for Disease Control and Prevention (CDC)—whereas other epidemiology research may employ retrospective review of medical, public health, and/or other records. Because epidemiology research often involves aggregate examination of data, it may not always be necessary to obtain individually identifiable information. When this is the case, the research may qualify for exemption or expedited review. You must provide the IRB with the proposal for the board to determine if IRB approval is required. There is often a form for expedited review and for exemption.
5. *Repository research.* Research that uses stored data or materials (cells, tissues, fluids, and body parts) from individually identifiable living or dead persons qualifies as human subject research and requires IRB review. When data or materials are stored in a bank or repository for use

in future research, the IRB should review a protocol that details the repository's policies and procedures for obtaining, storing, and sharing its resources; for verifying informed consent provisions; and for protecting subjects' privacy and maintaining the confidentiality of data. The IRB may then determine the parameters within which the repository may share its data or materials with or without IRB review of individual research protocols.

6. *Quality assurance activities.* Quality assurance activities attempt to measure the effectiveness of programs or services. Such activities may constitute human subject research and require IRB review if they are designed or intended to contribute to generalizable knowledge. Quality assurance activities that are designed solely for internal program evaluation purposes with no external application or generalization may not require IRB review. Again, the IRB must review the project to see if such activities require full IRB application and approval.

7. *Pilot studies.* Pilot studies that involve human subjects are considered human subject research and require IRB review.

The ethical conduct of research is a shared responsibility. It requires cooperation, collaboration, and trust among the institution, investigators, and their research staff; the subjects who enroll in research; and the IRBs. A clear delineation of the responsibilities of each of these parties can help protect the participants who volunteer for research.

RESPONSIBILITIES OF THE RESEARCH TEAM

The principal investigator (PI) is the individual responsible for the implementation of research and bears direct responsibility for protecting every research subject. This responsibility starts with protocol design, which must minimize risks to subjects while maximizing research benefits. In addition, the PI and all members of the research team must comply with the findings, determinations, and requirements of the IRB. The PI must also be responsible for the adequacy of both the informed consent document and the informed consent process, regardless of which members of the research team actually obtain and document consent.

Principal investigators have the following responsibilities: to ensure that all human subject research that they conduct in a particular institution or as employees or agents of that institution has received prospective review and approval by an IRB designated by the institution; that continuing review and approval of the research have been secured in a timely fashion; and that the research is conducted at all times in compliance with all applicable regulatory requirements and the determinations of the designated IRB. No changes in approved research may be initiated without prior IRB approval, except when necessary to eliminate apparent immediate hazards to subjects, and no research may be continued beyond the IRB-designated approval period. Investigators must notify the IRB promptly of any unanticipated problems or serious adverse events that involve risks to subjects or others, and any serious or continuing noncompliance with applicable regulatory requirements or determinations of the designated IRB of which they become aware.

Every member of the research team is responsible for protecting human subjects. Coinvestigators, study coordinators, nurses, research assistants, and all other research staff have a strict obligation to comply with all IRB determinations and procedures, adhere rigorously to all protocol requirements, inform investigators of all adverse subject reactions or unanticipated problems, oversee the adequacy of the informed consent process, and take whatever measures are necessary to protect the safety and welfare of subjects. Researchers at every level are responsible for notifying the IRB promptly of any serious or continuing noncompliance with applicable regulatory requirements or determinations of the designated IRB of which they become aware, regardless of whether they themselves are involved in the research.

Research subjects have responsibilities as well. They can be expected to make every effort to comprehend the information that researchers present to them so that they can make an informed decision about their participation in good faith. They should also be willing to comply with protocol requirements (unless they decide to discontinue participation) and inform the investigators of unanticipated problems. The OHRP assurances described previously require that research investigators receive appropriate initial and continuing education in the protection of human subjects. In addition, the National Institutes of Health (NIH) requires that all "key personnel" involved in NIH-supported human subject research receive training in protecting subjects. Check your institution's Web site for training in human subject protection. The NIH has a training program available on its Web site as well.

Some agencies—pharmaceutical companies, for example—may employ a contract research organization (CRO) to assist in preparing documents for IRB approval. You may partner with a CRO, provide your institution's IRB application and consent form template, and assist in the completion and/or review of the application before it is submitted to the local IRB. These agencies must comply with institutional requirements, and the application must be accompanied by a written agreement that specifies the responsibilities of the organization.

Generally, it is the study coordinator who completes the IRB application for review by the PI and then by the IRB. A study coordinator is one type of clinical research coordinator (CRC). According to the Association of Clinical Research Professionals, a CRC, regardless of job title, works at a clinical research site under the immediate direction of a PI, whose research activities are conducted under Good Clinical Practice (GCP) Guidelines. CRCs typically perform tasks such as:

- Site preparation
- Patient screening and recruitment
- Patient enrollment
- Conducting study visits
- Maintaining and dispensing drug supplies
- Completing and ensuring the quality of case report forms
- Maintaining source documents
- Ensuring site quality (2008)

THE IRB APPLICATION

The first place to begin an IRB application is your local institution's Web site. The IRB will have blank forms available for you to download and complete. It is very important that you have the most recent version of the proposal or protocol so that you can pull information from the proposal to complete the application. In addition, it is important to verify that you have the most recent version of the IRB template and consent form template.

There are directions for completing each of the sections. Use the proposal or the protocol and summarize each answer on the IRB application. There are a number of sections that relate to the principles discussed earlier. Generally, you will begin with information about the PI, followed by key personnel involved in the study (coinvestigators, study coordinator, research nurse, data coordinator, and biostatistician). Information about the duration of the project, the number of research participants or subjects, how you will recruit these participants, age and gender of the participants, and funding for the project needs to be provided. It is also important to the IRB that the PI have appropriate experience to lead the study. A curriculum vitae (CV) and/or a biosketch (for NIH or Department of Defense contracts) should be amended to the application.

Information about the type of study is also required. If it is a new drug or device project, you will append the IND or the IDE and place the corresponding number from the FDA on the application. Amend the investigator's brochure to the application.

There are also questions related to the use of biohazard materials or the use of devices on research participants. Prior to submitting the application, meet with individuals from radiation safety or biomedical engineering so that these departments can verify that you are safely using isotopes or machinery. Many IRBs require that a separate letter from these departments go directly to the IRB as a supplement to the application.

THE MEAT OF THE RESEARCH

Now to the meat of the research: The next section in the application allows you to discuss hypotheses, study design, treatments, importance of the research, and risks and benefits to the participants.

Because the IRB is ultimately concerned with safety, the establishment of a data safety monitoring board (DSMB) is a vital part of the application. The PI can establish the board for a biomedical research project. The DSMB members constitute an independent group of experts in the research and treatment of individuals with conditions being studied in the protocol. The board agrees to meet early with quarterly conference calls to discuss the course of participant involvement in the study. The DSMB also reviews any adverse events and helps decide if a project should continue or if the project should be suspended pending changes.

Another section involves reporting adverse events and additional safety information—in particular, who can be contacted in the event that a participant requires assistance. If a participant wishes to withdraw from the study, specific steps must be detailed.

Another very important piece of the research project is the informed consent document (ICD). The consent form contains a number of headings, including the following: General Info, Purpose, Information about Study Subjects, What Happens to Subjects in the Study, Risks/Benefits, Other Choices if a Patient Does Not Wish to Participate in Research, How to End Participation in the Study, Financial Information, Confidentiality/PHI (protected health information), Contact Information, Record of Information Provided, and Signatures. When writing a consent form, it is important to keep the language at an eighth-grade level. There are helpful tools online to assess the grade level of the consent form. Microsoft Office has a tool called the Flesch-Kincaid Grade Level that can be used to evaluate the reading level of the consent form. Another tip is to have a layperson review the consent form to assess ease of reading and understanding of the form.

When outlining the risks and benefits, you may need to note that the benefit may be to society, or it may be to the participants or others at a later time. Reviewing costs or payments to the participants is important. Outline for the participants when and how they will receive payment(s), especially if prorated. Emphasize time commitments, especially for more involved studies. In addition, state that participants may need to let their healthcare provider know that they are involved in research. Explain "randomization" concepts, especially if subjects may not receive the study treatment. Industry may want specific language included; review with the IRB if this may be added or modified in the consent form. The consent process is rarely a one-time event; it should continue throughout the subject's entire participation on a study.

Use your resources. Some IRBs have application specialists to help ensure that you have completed all necessary parts of the application. There may also be a scientific specialist to review the science. Find a colleague who has successfully received IRB approval and ask him or her to help you or review your application.

Make sure you know what is expected of you in the future as far as the IRB is concerned. Your relationship with the IRB is not over with the initial application. There are yearly updates and a final close-out report. But don't close out too soon; even if you're closed to enrollment, you may still be collecting and/or analyzing data and will need to keep the project "open" with the IRB. A final tip: Review what you'll need to report in your annual review so that you are sure that you are collecting that data from the start. For example, the NIH requirements include statistics on gender, ethnicity, and age; assure collection of this information on a deidentified case report form.

As you compile documents for your IRB application, you may need to include a research budget. Remember to budget for the IRB review. Check your institution's Web site; the review can be thousands of dollars.

Now you are ready to submit the application. Complete a cover page that explains what you are submitting and include who may be contacted if the IRB has any questions. Keep your fingers crossed and good luck!

Possible attachments:

☐ CV and/or biosketches
☐ HIPAA certificate for key personnel
☐ Case report forms (CRFs)
☐ Survey instruments
☐ Scripts
☐ Pathology forms delineating lab value ranges
☐ Budgets

☐ Investigational drug pharmacy application
☐ Conflict of interest and financial disclosure statements
☐ Investigational brochure
☐ Recruitment notices or advertisements
☐ Informed consent document(s)
☐ Grant application

Helpful Web sites:

For Human Subjects Training (National Institutes of Health):
http://www.nih.gov

A Tour of the FDA:
http://www.eduneering.com/fda/courses/fdatour/welcome.html

Overview of Drug Development Processes:
http://www.fda.gov/cder/handbook

DHHS, Department of Health and Human Services:
http://www.hhs.gov

DHHS Office for Human Research Protections (OHRP):
http://www.hhs.gov/ohrp
http://www.hhs.gov/ohrp/humansubjects/guidance/45cfr46.htm

REFERENCES

Association of Clinical Research Professionals. (2008). *CRC definition.* FDA CRC Certification Guide (North America)—March 2009. Retrieved November 19, 2008, from http://216.147.199.31/PDF/FDA-CRC-Guide.pdf

U.S. Department of Health and Human Services. (1979). *The Belmont Report.* Office for Human Research Protections (OHRP). Retrieved November 19, 2008, http://www.hhs.gov/ohrp/humansubjects/guidance/belmont.htm

U.S. Department of Health and Human Services. (1998). *Part 56 — Institutional Review Boards.* Code of Federal Regulations [21CFR 56.107(e)]. Retrieved November 19, 2008, from http://www.accessdata.fda.gov/scripts/cdrh/cfdocs/cfCFR/CFRSearch.cfm?fr=56.107

U.S. Department of Health and Human Services. (1999). *Part 5 — Freedom of Information Regulations.* Code of Federal Regulations [45CFR 46.103]. Retrieved November 19, 2008, from http://www.hhs.gov/foia/45cfr5.html

CHAPTER 7

Passage Through the Divide

Shelley Thibeau

*This chapter begins the "real stories of nursing research" as told by our contributor colleagues.

The year 2002 was a turning point in my nursing career. Our neonatal intensive care unit (NICU) became a member of a continuous quality improvement collaborative. During a Web-based series that focused on reducing nosocomial (now referred to as "hospital acquired") infections, I was exposed to continuous quality improvement tools, such as cycles for change using the plan, do, check, and act (PDCA) model; performance audits; and various methods to chart outcomes over time. Change management, the ability to impact patient care by motivating others to use current evidence in practice, became an exciting new career option.

As I began to research advanced educational opportunities, I discovered the health systems management master of science in nursing curriculum, which offered the necessary change management tools to successfully promote quality patient care. I enrolled in the fall of 2005 as an adult learner working full time. The return to nursing theory and nursing leadership concepts was a pleasurable experience. Nursing research and continuous quality improvement courses helped clarify the process of the knowledge transfer of evidence-based practice to bedside care. I realized that performance improvement is the process to improve patient outcomes, whereas research is the systematic inquiry into discovering new knowledge that can then be applied to processes used to improve patient outcomes. This is when the research world captured my interest; hence, I chose to shadow a nurse researcher for the practicum/clinical requirement of the master's program. Out of my comfort zone, I followed this mentor for over 300 hours to learn about her role within our organization. It was amazing to learn of the various projects within our organization that sought her expertise, each using the interplay of disciplines to achieve better outcomes.

The nurse researcher role appeared to be the conduit for nursing to bring evidence-based practice to bedside care. It became clear that the translation of relevant research into best practices was not a skill easily acquired at the bedside, yet the desire to improve practice was universal among many of our nurses. To explore this gap, I chose to conduct a literature search examining the integration of evidence-based practice into bedside nursing care as the capstone of the master of nursing program. The literature revealed various strategies that have reported success in mentorship models designed to accelerate evidence-based practice integration.

One of the organization's strategic goals was the development of a clinical scholar program to mentor a core group of bedside clinicians in evidence-based practice skills. Curriculum development for this program required a needs assessment of nurses' readiness for evidence-based practice. With mentor guidance, I embarked on a descriptive exploratory research study designed to assess our nurses' readiness for evidence-based practice, which was completed in two short months. The measurement instrument used was a modified survey derived from a national study. Permission was obtained from the original author by the mentor; the mentor also provided guidance through the approval process within our organization, to include a nursing research committee review and an institutional review board application. This proved to be an ideal way to experience the research process without feeling overwhelmed. The findings of the survey were analyzed by an in-house statistician; interpretation was again guided by the mentor. Results of the survey will direct curriculum development and planning of a nursing scholar program.

Experiencing the research process with a knowledgeable mentor confirmed my desire to facilitate change in nursing knowledge and practice. Research mentors placed in clinical settings are the key to bridging the divide that separates academia from bedside practice. As we close this knowledge gap with nursing scholar programs, more nurses will feel empowered to observe, analyze, evaluate, and change practice to improve patient outcomes. This should result in increased nursing autonomy and self-actualization.

Acknowledgment: The author would like to recognize and thank Dr. Karen Rice for the key role that she played as a positive mentor in the author's world of research.

Assessing Nurses' Readiness for Evidence-Based Practice

Shelley Thibeau, MSN, RNC;
and Karen L. Rice, DNSc, APRN, BC

Purpose: The purpose of this study was to conduct a needs assessment of nurses' readiness for evidence-based practice. Results will direct curriculum development for a nursing scholars program designed to promote the integration of evidence-based practice into bedside nursing care.

Design: A descriptive exploratory design was used to survey evidence-based practice awareness and learning needs of nurses employed at an academic tertiary care facility.

Methods: The instrument used for the survey was a 30-item questionnaire with reported satisfactory face and content validity, and internal consistency reliability. Data collection was completed using an Internet-accessible survey available to all nurses for a 1-month period. Data analysis included descriptive statistics and chi-square analysis to test for differences between demographic groups and survey items, $\alpha = 0.05$.

Results: A total of 180 of 1,200 (15%) nurses responded. Demographics revealed that the majority of respondents were staff nurses (88.9%), female (96.7%), and baccalaureate prepared (56.4%). Chi-square testing for differences between demographic groups found 15 variables to be statistically significant ($p < 0.05$). Younger nurses were more likely to ask a peer for information ($p = 0.006$), whereas older nurses were more likely to seek information from peer-reviewed journals ($p = < 0.001$) and conferences ($p = < 0.001$). Experienced nurses reported more participation in research ($p = 0.012$) and identification of potential areas of research ($p = 0.019$). Tenured nurses reported increased participation ($p = 0.013$), evaluation ($p = 0.038$), and identification of areas for research ($p = 0.019$). The majority of respondents identified lack of compensated time as the greatest barrier to evidence-based practice (70.6%) and listed lack of knowledge about evidence-based practice (41.7%) as the second most predominant barrier. Improving patient care was perceived as a personal goal in using research to guide nursing practice for the majority of respondents (80.7%).

Conclusion: The survey respondents identified knowledge management, such as skills in the use of bibliographic databases and skills in critical appraisal of the literature and translation into practice, as lacking competencies for evidence-based practice integration. Nurses identified lack of compensated time as a barrier to integration of evidence-based practice into bedside care but recognized support services for integration of evidence-based practice within the organization and support by nursing leadership. Results support the inclusion of content that targets strategies to address learning needs of the bedside nurse as identified in this study. A nursing scholar program composed of a skills lab and mentored practicum is expected to accelerate evidence-based practice integration into bedside nursing care.

(2007)

CHAPTER 8

It's All About Inquiry!

Mary Beth Leaton

So you're reading this book because you're looking for some insight into, advice about, and perhaps wisdom for carrying out your first nursing research study. First let me applaud you and thank you for your commitment to nursing. Now let me ask you some questions. Are you the type of person who, when out to dinner with friends, finds yourself asking the "big philosophical life questions" that cause your spouse or friends to roll their eyes? After watching a movie, do you feel compelled to analyze the meaning behind the movie? When you are in a clinical setting, do you constantly wonder what the best way to manage a patient is? If you answered "yes" to any of these questions, then you have the essential characteristics of a researcher: that of inquiry. Inquiry is simply part of who you are. This characteristic surfaced early in my life. At a young age, to my parents' shock, I took apart the family TV because I wanted to know how it worked. Luckily, both my parents are teachers, and my father was handy with a screwdriver. Despite my curious nature, I was a late bloomer with regard to carrying out my first research study.

I attended my undergraduate program from 1984 to 1988, and although research was part of the program, the message was clear: Research was carried out by doctoral-prepared academic faculty. I left my undergraduate program after learning how to analyze and discuss a concept, and how nursing theories are generated and tested. After graduation, I never wanted to see another library card catalog and appreciated the incredible value of a helpful librarian. So, although I enjoyed the academic discussions around research in my undergraduate program, I did not make a connection with nursing research and the clinical setting. It all seemed very abstract and, well, theoretical. There were no discussions of evidence-based practice, and the closest I came to evidence-based practice was including the references for my care plans. Back then, CINAHL (Cumulative Index to Nursing and Allied Health Literature) was a set of bound books in the library, and the concept of searching a database online was in its infancy.

I started my nursing career during a nursing shortage and was accepted into an internship program for critical care. Critical care was a perfect fit for my curious mind. It is a setting that expects you to know every detail regarding your patient and to constantly ask questions about what is going on with him or her. The hospital I started in was a community teaching facility, so we had medical resident teaching rounds, although nursing was not really part of those rounds at that time (how far we have come!). I took advantage of the opportunity to learn. What I found very interesting was that the medical residents were expected to be able to cite references regarding their treatment recommendations during patient rounds. At the time, this was not an expectation for nurses. My preceptors and educators focused on what the policy and procedure manual said—there were no discussions regarding best practices. As I continued my nursing career in critical care, I came to a point where my "need to know more" surfaced again. I thought that going back to graduate school to become a clinical nurse specialist (CNS) would help me become the clinical expert I truly wanted to be and improve my understanding of research. So I started graduate school in 1993.

My first class was statistics in the Department of Sociology, and it was excellent. The focus of the class was on understanding statistics rather than the formulas used to calculate statistical values. (I was very thankful, because mathematics makes me break out in hives.) The statistics software program we used was SPSS—not the Windows-based statistical program we use now, but a program that required us to write the code to execute the command. This was the bane of my graduate life because I have dyslexia, and writing computer codes would take me hours—but I got through it. Once again, my research classes included the analysis of concepts and development of nursing theories, but we also started to critique nursing studies. I understood how to write a review of the literature, identify the gaps in nursing knowledge, determine the appropriate study design to address the research question, and analyze the findings. It was at this point that I appreciated the basic building blocks of research that I gained in my undergraduate program. I began to make the connection between nursing theory and well-designed studies that would address clinical research questions. This was primarily due to one professor who led my clinical practicum seminar. She taught us how to search the literature, rate the literature, and then summarize the research findings. We were expected to be the expert on our chosen topic. She required us to use research studies or reviews of the literature to address the clinical questions we generated during our practicum. I am forever thankful for this professor.

Although I did not need to complete a research study in my graduate program, I did need to complete a research proposal. This process reinforced some of the basic research skills acquired during the program, but I did not feel prepared, in any manner, to be a primary investigator for a research study. The philosophy of the university I attended was that a master's degree was not a terminal degree; as such, we were taught how to be consumers of research but not necessarily expected to carry out a research study. So I left my graduate program able to critique an article, interpret a p value, and comprehend descriptive/correlation studies.

Fast forward seven years. I am a CNS for the critical care areas in a small community hospital. One day I find myself sitting in a nursing leadership meeting reviewing the criteria to achieve Magnet status. We came to the criterion for research, and the room became quiet. In the group of nursing leaders was a director for the medical/surgical division who had worked in an organization when it applied for Magnet designation. She proposed that we do a replication study of Dr. Linda Aiken's work on professional work environments. This was a brilliant idea. It would provide us with information regarding our nurses' perception of the practice environment and help us begin to meet the research requirement for Magnet designation. So, the next logical question for the group was: Who would take on the responsibility for this study? I looked at my "partner in crime," another CNS for oncology, and gave her a look like, "We have to do this, are you in?" In return, she gave me that "Are you out of your mind?" look. In the end, it was my partner in crime and I who were responsible for the study.

We felt totally overwhelmed. Although we both had an understanding of the basics, we were clueless when it came to creating a code book, entering data into a statistical program, and analyzing the data. As luck would have it, another CNS was working with a pediatric advanced nurse practitioner who was a faculty member at a local university. She was a PhD candidate at the time and graciously offered to help us with the study. I cannot express my gratitude enough for her help. She walked us through every step of the study, from the study design through analyzing the findings. It was a simple descriptive survey study, but it seemed like so much more to us. You would have thought we were carrying out a multicenter prospective double-blind randomized control study! Sadly, at the end of our study, there was a change in the hospital leadership, and the decision was made not to pursue Magnet designation. As we were in the process of interpreting and disseminating our results, the study was discontinued. Despite this anticlimactic ending, I am incredibly thankful for that experience because it ignited my passion for research and gave me a wee bit of confidence to pursue other studies.

Okay, let us fast forward again to 2006. Now I am the CNS for an ICU at a Magnet-designated teaching hospital, Morristown Memorial Hospital. I was sitting in a meeting of the Evidence Based Nursing Practice Committee. We had just completed a Magnet redesignation, and one of the two recommendations for growth by the surveyors was to create a more consistent culture of evidence-based nursing practice (EBNP) throughout the organization. The group was trying to create a plan for the year to address this recommendation. We talked about bringing in speakers, having workshops, and holding classes on EBNP. Although we had some good ideas, I felt we really needed to have some baseline data on where our nurses stood regarding EBNP.

Once again, a little bit of luck intervened; I had just read a study completed by Drs. Pravikoff, Tanner, and Pierce (2005) that was published in the *American Journal of Nursing*, titled "Readiness of U.S. Nurses for Evidence-Based Practice: Many don't understand or value research and have had little or no training to help them find evidence on which to base their practice." The study examined nurses' readiness to use EBNP and focused on the resources needed for EBNP and on the various computer literacy skills needed to access scientific literature. It was perfect timing. We could replicate this study as an assessment of our nurses and create a plan to support the development of EBNP in our organization. The group agreed. Unlike my last experience, this time I had a fairly good idea of how to proceed. I also had wonderful resources at this Magnet organization: a fantastic librarian, online access to databases, a faculty consultant, and a nurse researcher on site. How great is that! (As an aside, I feel compelled to mention that I think the ANCC's Magnet requirement for research has done a tremendous amount to evolve the development of clinical nursing research. The difference is phenomenal between what I have seen in Magnet and non-Magnet organizations regarding attitudes and resources committed to nursing research.) With their guidance and the help of two other nurses, we completed the study. Yes, it was a simple descriptive survey, but we did it from start to finish. We wrote the proposal, applied for IRB approval, stuffed hundreds of nursing mailboxes with surveys, entered what seemed like one million data points, analyzed the data, interpreted the results, and summarized our conclusions. At the same time we were carrying out our study, ONE-NJ also replicated the study throughout New Jersey. This was very reaffirming for us. When ONE-NJ had their research day to present their results, I was invited to present our results and the actions we had taken based on those findings. We used research to address a problem that the organization faced, and the results provided us with a systematic approach to analyze the issue.

After completing this study, I had a much better understanding of the logistics of carrying out a research study. I felt that research really could be applied to answer our questions in nursing. It no longer seemed so abstract and academic to me. I also never could have estimated how time consuming it was, and this was just a simple descriptive study. Because it had been many years since my statistics course, I had to go back to the textbooks and review the content. It is amazing how you develop a great motivation to reread those chapters on nonparametric versus parametric statistics when you are knee-deep in data! I think the other aspect of completing this study was the unexpected requests to present the study findings and how we used the results. I have been invited to speak at three local conferences on the topic of EBNP, which really emphasizes the importance of disseminating study results. Other organizations are faced with very similar issues. Simply stated, writing a proposal, or perhaps a systematic review of the literature, cannot compare to the personal experience and confidence gained in completing a study, no mater how simple the design.

The second study I was involved in was another replication study (replication studies are a novice researcher's best friend) that examined pain assessment in nonverbal ICU patients. Currently, I am coinvestigator for a study examining nurses' perceptions regarding fever. This study will serve as a basis for filling the gap in nursing knowledge regarding fever assessment and management and will be used in the development of an EBNP guideline for nursing fever management. So once again, I am finding the need to know more, and I feel the pull to enter a PhD program.

OK, so let's get back to why you are reading this book. After all, this is about your path in pursuing research, right? Let me share with you some of the lessons I have learned as a "late bloomer" in research. Start by jotting down your clinical questions or clinical problems facing your unit or organization. Pick one of those clinical questions or problems and become an expert on that topic. It is in this way that you will truly understand where the gaps exist in nursing knowledge regarding your topic of interest, and you will be able to write the literature review with ease. Remember, no one can ask your clinical research question but you! This will form the basis of where to begin planning your research study. Then find a research "buddy" who shares your passion. I always find new experiences easier to go through with a buddy or a partner in crime. Pick someone you have a good relationship with and who inspires you. I believe that when you put two inspired and determined nurses together, there is nothing that can't be accomplished.

Along the same lines, take stock of what your support and resources are to carry out your research study. It is incredibly important to find that support before you start your study. What is available to you? For example, do you have clinical faculty who have clinical rotations in your facility? Perhaps your nursing administration/education department meets with your local nursing programs. Consider discussing a collaborative relationship to start nursing research in your organization. I have found that faculty truly can be an invaluable support and will often donate their time because your facility is providing a clinical setting for their students. Do you have a biostatistician available to you, perhaps through the medical department? Do you have a medical department of research and access to a statistical program? Do you have a hospital foundation that may consider funding a nursing research consultant? Get to know your hospital librarian. Do you have a research committee? Perhaps research is already being conducted in your organization. If so, go and talk to those individuals and offer your time to help with the study. If you are a graduate student, take advantage of a research assistantship, if offered. Any experience gained in the research process is well worth it. Talk to your facility's leadership about carrying out research investigations and gain their support for the research process.

Choosing your first research study can be overwhelming. My advice is to keep it simple, and replication studies with a "twist" are a great way to start. Replicating a study with some slight variation is a good way to get your first research experience. Oftentimes, the original study's author(s) will be more than happy to guide you through replicating their study. Choose a topic that will meet a specific need for your unit or organization. This will often give you administrative support and time to carry out your study. By choosing a study topic in which data collection can be integrated into your daily routine, you will be more successful in staying committed to the study.

There is so much more I would like to share, but I think the best way to overcome your fear of nursing research is simply to do it. No study is too simple if it answers a clinically important question and is well designed. Any experience gained is invaluable, and something you will certainly build on. If you have passion for clinical inquiry, you will succeed. I wish you all the best on your research path and thank you for making a difference in the care we provide our patients.

Acknowledgment: I'd like to extend my deepest gratitude to the following colleagues who have supported me on my research journey: Dr. Carole Birdsall, Dr. Jane Dillert, Maureen Fitzsimmons, Denise Fochesto, and Dr. Susan Fowler. Their guidance, encouragement, and witty insights kept me sane and focused on my research journey.

Readiness of Nurses at a Community Teaching Hospital to Use Evidence-Based Practice

Mary Beth Leaton, MS, RN, CCRN, APN;
Sherry (Sharon) Ninni, BSN, RN, CCRN; and Janet Munoz, BSN, RN

Introduction: A recent study published by Pravikoff and colleagues (2005) identified that in a sample of 760 RNs, only 46% were familiar with the term *evidence-based practice*, and 67% of respondents never searched the CINAHL database. They concluded that RNs in the United States are not ready for evidence-based practice because of the gaps in their information literacy and computer skills, limited access to high-quality information resources, and, above all, the attitudes of nurses and nursing administrators toward research. The purpose of this study was to replicate Pravikoff, et al.'s study to determine the information literacy needs regarding evidence-based practice of the RNs at Morristown Memorial Hospital (MMH).

Methods: A total of 1,100 surveys were distributed to MMH nurses. A total of 227 (or 20.6%) surveys were returned.

Results: Eighty-one percent of MMH nurses were familiar with the term *evidence-based practice (EBP)*, as opposed to 46% of nurses in the national survey. Thirty-four percent of nurses were participating in a journal club. Sixty percent of respondents rated the print and online resources as adequate or more then adequate. Fifty-six percent of respondents have engaged in some aspect of research two to three times this year, versus 46.6% in the national survey. The majority of MMH nurses seek information from reference texts (79%) or journals (73%), as opposed to seeking information from research articles (10%) or the hospital library (0%). When respondents were asked, "When you need information, how do you find it?" the majority of respondents most frequently asked a peer (52%) and searched the Internet (39%). There was a statistically significant difference between certified and noncertified nurses, with certified nurses (1) seeking information from journals ($p = .000$) and CINAHL ($p = .001$) more frequently and (2) being familiar with the term *EBP* ($p = .002$). There was a significant difference among nurses based on their level of education, with master's-prepared nurses seeking information from journals (p = .002), research (p = .001), and CINAHL (p = .001) more frequently. Nurses who participated in journal clubs were five times more likely to seek information from a journal or an electronic database, and 10 times more likely to seek information from the Web than those nurses who did not participate in a journal club.

Discussion: MMH nurses had similar findings to the national survey regarding the frequency with which they needed information for their role and the resources they used for their information. MMH nurses differed from the national survey in that a greater percentage of nurses were familiar with the term *EBP* and had participated in some aspect of research.

Implications: Based on the findings of this study, an action plan was devised to (1) increase the number of online nursing journals/reference books, (2) bring the librarian to the unit for educational sessions on electronic databases and EBP resources, (3) develop a quick reference nursing EBP Web page, (4) support nursing certification, and (5) increase the number of unit-based journal clubs.

REFERENCES

Pravikoff, D. S., Tanner, A. B., & Pierce, S. T. (2005). Readiness of U.S. nurses for evidence-based practice: Many don't understand or value research and have had little or no training to help them find evidence on which to base their practice. *American Journal of Nursing 105*(9), 40–51.

CHAPTER 9

Stepping Out of the Box into the Sphere of Research

Sandra Marconi

When someone mentioned research, the first thing that used to come to my mind was doctors working in a lab and discovering the cure for some disease. I came to Penn State Hershey Medical Center (PSHMC) 15 years ago and started working on the pediatric inpatient unit. Two years ago, my nurse educator challenged me and other members of our nursing education council to come out of our box and become involved in research. She gave us the goal of writing an article about our work and getting it published. I have been a registered nurse since 1975, and before coming to PSHMC, no one had ever encouraged me to do any research. It was a challenge that I accepted.

I was thrilled to become involved with this project. With over 30 years of nursing experience, I have witnessed the increased need for continuing education. These requirements are necessary in some states not only to meet regulatory requirements, such as relicensure, but also for professional growth and development. I wanted to be involved in helping my colleagues with learning experiences that were meaningful to their nursing responsibilities.

I had been active on the nursing education council for several years. Our nursing education council was responsible for identifying the learning needs of our staff nurses and in conducting competency checks related to the use of patient care equipment. Many times, the review of skills and knowledge was for complex patient care equipment that was used infrequently. When we first started the training, it took less than 30 minutes to verify each nurse's skill in using the equipment. With the development of new equipment and new therapies, the required training and testing time had increased to well over an hour for each nurse. Our education council members discussed the issue and decided as a group that there was a need to identify which competencies were important to keep and which could be modified or eliminated. We recognized that it was essential to make these decisions without compromising the quality of patient care and safety.

Each year, members of our education council would test other staff nurses on their competency in the use of specialized equipment through review and test methods. During our council meeting, we discussed whether the staff retained the information from year to year, how they progressed in their learning, and if the training met new learning needs. We also wanted to identify specifically which pieces of equipment the staff were competent in using so that we could modify and/or replace those competency areas with others for the following year to ensure effective learning. In addition, we needed to encourage teamwork to help meet the increasing demands for education.

The decision was made to develop a listing of each subskill that could be used to document competency for each skill. Competency completion without cueing from the council member was documented with a plus sign, and competency with cueing from the council member was documented with a minus sign. The data were collected and entered into a spreadsheet. After our yearly competencies were completed, we reviewed the gathered information. Based on the data, the group identified three competencies that could be eliminated for the next year and one that could be modified. One new competency was identified and added to the next year's list. This systematic review of our data told us that our nursing research was a success. We wanted to share this news with others, so the council members decided that our facilitator would write the article that we would submit for publication. After the first draft was written, she sent it to each council member. We were responsible for reading and editing it, and returning our suggestions to her. Everyone's opinion was valued. Each council member reviewed the article once again before submitting it for publication. To our great surprise, our article was accepted for publication in the *Journal for Nurses in Staff Development*.

Through doing this research, I have gained the confidence to take on more responsibility in my current position. I work in the pediatric stem cell transplant clinic, where I am responsible for preparing the clinic sheets for the physicians, checking in patients to the clinic, doing vital signs, reviewing medications, and drawing blood for tests. Because the nurse specialist resigned, I am usually the only nurse in the clinic. I review the lab results with the physicians and families. For tests that take longer than the average time to obtain results, I notify the physician so that medication changes can be made in a timely manner if needed. I call the families with the changes. I am also responsible for infusions that the stem cell patients need, such as IVIG platelets, packed red blood cells, cidofovir, and pentamidine. I also do enzyme replacement for patients with Fabray disease, Pompee disease, Hunter's syndrome, and Hurler's syndrome. Two of these enzymes were approved by the FDA less then two years ago. Rheumatology patients also receive their remicade infusions in the clinic where I work.

In my position, I meet with the pediatric stem cell transplant team every week. Once a month, a member of the team presents a research article and shares the findings with the other members. As expected and with some apprehension, I took my turn in this shared learning experience. I read several research articles before I decided on the article "Bone Marrow Donation: Factors Influencing Intentions in African Americans." I presented the article at our October 2007 meeting. I was greatly encouraged by the discussion of the group after I presented the article. We talked about ways that we could increase the national bone marrow registry for African Americans and other minorities. It is more difficult to find matches for African Americans and other minorities than it is for Caucasians, whose registry is larger. Because of this deficit, some patients die waiting for a stem cell transplant because we are unable to find a match. I plan on presenting another research article in 2008. I know that I will be active in doing literature searches for the best available evidence and in participating in research when asked.

I have taken on other new roles and responsibilities since coming to Penn State Children's Hospital (PSCH). When the pediatric stem cell transplant program was first started at PSCH, I had no interest in being involved. I soon realized that this was a new area in nursing that offered a professional opportunity for me. Some of my patients would not survive without a transplant. While working on the inpatient unit, I developed interdisciplinary education records to use in teaching stem cell transplant patients and their families. At the same time, I became active in organizing stem cell transplant classes for new nurses, an activity I continue today. I developed a stem cell transplant glossary for the stem cell transplant clinic and the inpatient unit. A year ago, I became a Pediatric Advanced Life Support Instructor. I instruct other nurses, residents, physicians, respiratory therapists, and EMTs. Through this work, I discovered the recent research for more effective cardio-pulmonary resuscitation. This firsthand experience using the research literature led me to understand that nurses are involved in research more than many of us realize.

As an active member of the Association of Pediatric Hematology/Oncology Nurses, I attend educational meetings throughout the year. With this group, I am able to share and learn about new patient care and treatments, including new therapies for pediatric cancer patients and sickle cell patients. These experiences have given me the confidence and skills to work on cutting-edge treatments that make a difference to patients. For example, I have administered a special experimental drug to stem cell patients who had developed veno-occlusive disease. The drug is not yet approved by the FDA, so our physicians had to obtain permission to import this drug from Italy. Working under appropriate protocols and within the scope of nursing practice, I was one of the nurses who administered the drug and saw firsthand the positive response that patients had to this treatment. It was exciting for me to be part of research that has had such a positive effect on patient outcomes.

When I first became a nurse, children diagnosed with cancer were handed a death sentence. Now, the cure for all types of cancer has an amazing 90% success rate. Fifteen years ago, pediatric patients with acute myeloid leukemia (AML) usually died. Many are now surviving after receiving a stem cell transplant. With all the medical advances and new therapies, I am one nurse who can no longer sit on the sidelines and not become involved. I believe it is our duty as nurses to provide the highest level of quality care for our patients. One of the best ways we can do this is by becoming active participants in research at all levels. When I first became a nurse, I never thought that I would be involved in research. Fear of the unknown is often what keeps us from leaving that which is familiar, and stepping into unfamiliar territory was not part of my comfort zone. I am grateful to my mentors, teachers, and colleagues who have helped me expand the sphere of possibilities in nursing research.

Acknowledgment: I would like to acknowledge Tara Jankouskas, the nurse educator who organized the research. She has been a great friend and resource.

Annual Competencies Through Self-Governance and Evidence-Based Learning

Tara Jankouskas, MSN, RN,C;
Renee Dugan, BSN, RN,C; Tracy Fisher, RN,C; Kathryn Freeman, RN;
Sandra Marconi, RN,C; Heather Miller, BSN, RN,C; Barbara Smith, BSN,
RN,C; Brandy Souders, BSN, RN; and Dolores Zoller, BSN, RN,C

Purpose: The staff nurse has increasing educational demands. The goal of this project was to identify the essential competencies needed by the staff nurses. This approach to annual competencies, along with evidence-based learning, builds teamwork. This teamwork promotes learning. Teamwork and competent nursing care leads to improved patient outcomes.

Design: The educational needs for the nursing staff were identified by the nursing education council members. Competencies were developed for each of the identified learning needs by the council members. Identified competencies included the resuscitation cart, the peritoneal dialysis machine, the insulin pen, the patient-controlled analgesia pump, chest tubes, the urimeter, the externalized ventricular shunt, and the apnea monitor. The council members identified a list of four to six subskills or knowledge of each competency. The clinical nurse educator reviewed all chosen competencies and related policies in detail with the education council. During the time that the staff nurse attended the 1-hour competency education, the clinical nurse educator supported the competency training by providing coverage for patient care.

Methods: The education council members chose a learning method of return demonstration. Each staff nurse demonstrated actual use of the listed skills for each piece of equipment in order to show competency. A council member guided and watched over this demonstration. Data were collected on the ability of each nurse to complete each subskill for each competency. An Excel spreadsheet was used to document competency for each skill. Each competency that was completed without cueing from the council member was documented with a plus sign. If the staff nurse needed assistance, it was documented with a minus sign. If the nurse was unable to complete the skill or perform it correctly, the council member properly demonstrated the skill and reviewed the related policy and procedure.

Results and Conclusions: The patient-controlled analgesia competency and all the subskills were demonstrated without cueing for 94–98% of the staff nurses. The educational council agreed to delete this competency based on the data. The council decided to replace it with a new competency on preparing complex intravenous lines. The nurses demonstrated a competency of 93–95% on all subskills except for the skill for collecting a specimen, which had a competency rating of 84%. The council modified this competency to one skill. The insulin pin had one subskill, priming of the pin, with a rating greater than 90%. This subskill was deleted. The subskill of checking chest tubes for air leaks also scored greater than 90%. Therefore, the council deleted this subskill. Staff provided positive feedback after participating in the annual competency review. They valued the opportunity to review the annual competencies through skill demonstration, and they valued the opportunity to ask questions in a nonthreatening atmosphere. Education council members often serve as the expert resource for questions or problems related to the complex pieces of equipment. In summary, a team environment was created that combined a self-governance approach with evidence-based learning. The goals of competent nursing practice and teamwork led to improved patient care and outcomes.

CHAPTER 10

From Overwhelmed and Lost to Published

Susan E. Powers

Research—how do you grasp it and find time to run with it? My first encounter with research was in graduate school. I was required to take a course. We learned the terminology and received a statistics computer package. I walked away overwhelmed and lost. In my job, there never seemed to be time to explore an idea of interest or concern. The statistics and probability information did not make a whole lot of sense.

In 2002, Winchester Hospital started its Magnet journey for recognition as having excellence in nursing. One of the requirements was to have four nursing councils. Research was one of the councils. My department director was assigned the task of setting up the research council and overseeing the research projects. She worked with the hospital institutional review board (IRB) and provided encouragement and support to all the nurses interested in research. We met on a regular basis and studied the book *The Essentials of Nursing Research* together. Through this process, I was able to learn and understand the terminology. We looked at research articles and critiqued them based on research-related criteria. A simple form was created that we used as a template to gather information. Everything was kept very simple. Soon we were looking at different places within our hospital where we wanted to provide evidence-based practice.

I was working on the creation and implementation of the Family Caregiver Program. This program was an addition to the Nurse Aide Training Program that I had created several years earlier. We applied for grant funding to pilot the program. My department director asked me one simple question: How would I like to do a research project with the program? My first reaction was that it was not big enough to do research on. Then I said, "Why me? I do not have the time, and this is way too complex for me. I do not know how to do research." But I also knew that she and the team would work on this with me and that I would have a wonderful learning experience.

The number of elders requiring at-home care is increasing as our population ages. The healthcare system is able to manage chronic illness so that people live longer, thereby extending the time that families and the formal system must provide care. Although caregivers play a major role in assisting ailing or recovering senior family members at home, many do not know what kind of care is needed or how to provide it. Often they have no community or family resources to help them or give them a break from caregiving. Their role is demanding both physically and mentally, and there are few resources available to support and train them in the skills required.

Patients are often discharged after a short and intense hospital stay. There is not time to train the family caregivers and ensure that they are confident with the skills needed. The opportunity for research was present when we ran our first grant-funded Family Caregiver Program. We were able to evaluate the participants' confidence in providing the skills needed to care for their family member before they took the course and after they took the course.

I was excited that I was being given the opportunity to conduct a research project and that I would have the support I needed each step of the way. This was a great and rewarding challenge for me. I have always wanted to continue to learn new things for my stimulation and growth. Being able to prove that what I believed was correct was wonderful! Once I had actually been through the process, I realized how it worked. Looking for information through the literature search was very interesting. I was able to find out what others were learning about family caregivers and the work they were doing everywhere in the world. It really is quite simple if you take your hypothesis and follow the steps of the nursing research process.

I learned that nothing is too small or too insignificant to look at. The research I conducted was a pilot program with only 11 participants, and yet the results were statistically significant.

For me, the support and team effort made it work. The monthly research council meetings were a great help. We continue to look at research, discuss other staff members' research, and find that we are not alone.

When you write a paper or start a project, the hardest part is always getting the first sentence down on paper. The same is true with research. Once you have a doable hypothesis, you are off and running. It is easier to do research on your particular practice and interests. You will be able to provide better care with evidence-based practice that you identify. You will learn what works and what does not work. Evidence-based practice is very compelling.

Be sure you have the support and tools you need to do the research project. Find someone who can mentor you. Learn all the terminology. Create simple templates to follow for the research process and fill in the blanks. Become best friends with a library or librarian for your literature search. Find a statistician who will be supportive, explain things as you go along, and help you analyze the results.

Start small with something you know about. Bring your passion, interest, and knowledge to the table. Find something that you want to prove is right.

Embrace the literature research. You will find a lot that you did not know, and a lot that you know will be confirmed. Find out what has and has not already been done with your topic and hypothesis.

A replication study might be a good way to get started the first time. Search the literature regarding the subject of interest. I was able to have my research published in a professional journal. This was exciting because I have received calls from individuals who would like to replicate the study in two different countries!

Acknowledgment: The author would like to acknowledge the expertise of the nurse researcher Dr. Kathleen Beyerman for the guidance, patience, and expertise she provided to me as a novice researcher.

The Family Caregiver Program: A Pilot Study

Susan E. Powers, MS, RN

Purpose: To determine if the Family Caregiver Program, an educational intervention, is effective, we designed a quasi-experimental, quantitative pilot study to evaluate the impact of this educational program on caregivers' confidence in caregiving. The research question was: Does participation in the Family Caregiver Program increase feelings of confidence for caregivers in their caregiving skills? The hypothesis was: Family caregiver education will provide the knowledge that will increase the confidence level of the caregiver.

Design: The target population was family members caring for sick or recovering individuals who were over age 60. The convenience sample of 11 participants was gained through a variety of sources: the hospital's Senior Outreach Program, home care agencies, local senior centers, hospital staff, local churches, hospices, and self-referrals via press releases.

The two eligibility criteria were (1) the participant's ability to read and write English and (2) being the family caregiver of a patient aged 60 or older who was discharged from the hospital needing home care.

The age range of the caregiver participants was 45–84 years. Two of the participants worked outside the home, and 8 participants had a college education. Six of the participants lived with the family member for whom they provided care. All participants completed a demographic sheet and informed consent. The age range of the patients was 69–94 years. The patients were frail, and many of them had received care at home for more than a year. Their diagnoses and health problems included cellulitis, incontinence, immobility, obesity, end stage renal disease (dialysis), dementia, macular degeneration, progressive supra nuclear palsy, arthritis, depression, hearing loss, stroke, and Alzheimer's disease.

Methods: Study participants attended the Family Caregiver Program, which included 25 hours of classes. Nine of the participants attended every class; 2 attended all but one class. The reason for missing the classes was the need to take the person needing care to a medical appointment.

Results: There are 22 individual items on the Powers Elder Care Confidence Scale (PECCS). Thirteen of the 22 items showed a statistically significant difference between the pre- and posttest. The total mean score for the pretest was 3.5027, which is halfway between *undecided* and *agree*. The total mean score for the posttest was 4.2071, which is almost a whole point higher, and between *agree* and *strongly agree*. The training showed an improvement overall ($p > 0.002$). The posttest mean of 4.2071 is 22.8% higher than the pretest mean of 3.5027. This showed a 20–25% improvement in confidence due to the training.

An analysis of the pre and post difference in each item of the PECCS was completed. The items appeared to fall into two categories: (1) those items that were ranked highly at the beginning of the course and showed little room for improvement, and (2) those items that were initially ranked low and then improved with course participation. Items 1, 2, 20, and 21 on the PECCS pretest had a response of 4 or greater (5 being the highest ranking).

Conclusions: The study indicates that the Family Caregiver Program is effective in improving the confidence of the caregivers who participated in this education intervention. A formal training program provides caregivers with the knowledge and skills to better care for their elderly and ill family members. Winchester Hospital Community Health Institute plans to offer more Family Caregiver Programs with the support of the home care nurses. Nurses who provide formal education to caregivers will likely find that the care their patients receive meets patient needs and prevents rehospitalizations. Caregivers with more confidence in caregiving knowledge and skills can give better care to their loved ones!

(2002)

CHAPTER 11

A Different Way of Thinking: Using and Applying Evidence to Make Informed Decisions

Amy Hall McCowan

My current position as Director of Administration Projects at Penn State Milton S. Hershey Medical Center is not a title you will find in many hospitals. Honestly, it is a "home-grown" title that came along with a home-grown job description. I was a medical-surgical nurse turned nursing educator. I loved my job as a bedside nurse and as an educator. It gave me great satisfaction to care for patients and then educate other nurses about how to optimally care for their patients. I took my job very seriously and felt that I was in a position to make a direct impact on patient care in my role both as nurse educator and direct care nurse. When our chief nursing officer approached me about taking a job as a Director of Projects, I laughed. I never wanted to be far from clinical nursing, and a job in administration would do just that. It was not until I spoke with a nursing mentor of mine that I realized that there was such a need for nurses at the administrative level who understood grassroots nursing. This encounter is what prompted me to take my current position. I believed I could affect patient care and the well-being of nurses on a much larger scale if I chose to take my career to the next level. The many projects in which I have been involved include patient bed relocation for the medical center, selection of a nurse call system and wireless communication, and standardization of defibrillators.

Many of these projects come with information from the vendors that describes the advantages of their products. For me, the skeptical person that I am, I was always interested in asking, "Why?" So, not being satisfied that the vendor-supplied information and research were sufficient, I consulted the recent literature and my colleagues and nursing staff who would be using the equipment.

When I was asked to take on the issue of the dress code for nursing, it was an obvious choice for me to consult the literature. Admittedly, I have never been a true fan of conducting "research" (the word scares me). However, I realized that we would be operating in a bubble if we allowed ourselves to make selections purely based on opinion. Opinion is important, particularly when you are addressing how someone should dress, but there are other resources to consider—particularly when you are trying to capture how a patient would react to a particular uniform choice. Short of conducting our own patient survey, the literature was the next best thing! Getting the small group to buy into the literature findings had its challenges. The patient care assistants (PCAs) did not want to hear about what the literature suggested; they were interested, quite naturally, in seeing that their choices would be considered first and foremost. When confronted with the evidence, it was obvious that the PCAs needed to reconsider their views. After discussion, they realized that their preferences needed reevaluation in light of the support from the literature that reported that PCAs should not wear scrubs. This integration of best available evidence with the initial prevailing views and opinions of PCAs resulted ultimately in a best practice that was congruent with the original goals. The selected uniform was professional and functional and made the PCA easily identifiable to patients.

Using Best Available Evidence to Select Patient Care Assistant Uniforms

Amy McCowan, MEd, RN, CMSRN

Purpose: Whether you work at a fast food restaurant, have children who attend school, or volunteer at the local fire company, uniforms are a hot topic. In healthcare settings, this matter is an even more burning issue. It is crucial that hospitalized patients be able to identify the phlebotomist, housekeeper, or other ancillary person from their registered nurse. This project shows the process that the Penn State Milton S. Hershey Medical Center (PSHMC) used to evaluate and update the Department of Nursing's professional dress code as it relates to patient care assistants (PCAs).

Methods: For nearly 30 years, PCAs at PSHMC have worn identical uniforms provided by the institution. It became clear that the style of uniform they had been wearing for approximately the last 10 years was outdated and not work-friendly. A multidisciplinary group made up of nurse managers, human resource personnel, staff nurses, and PCAs joined forces to choose another type of uniform. The goals were clear: There was a crucial need to provide a work-friendly uniform (with pockets and made of a breathable fabric) that looked professional, and, most important, made the PCA easily identifiable to any patient or visitor. We started our project by surveying the 80 PCAs on staff. We asked questions about color choice and uniform choice, such as scrubs versus polo shirts and slacks, or another type of uniform. Members of the Nursing Quality of Work Life Council performed a literature search to determine the existing evidence and best practices.

Results: Responses from the PCA survey showed an overwhelming request for scrubs. Reports from the literature review suggested that patients identified healthcare workers wearing scrubs as registered nurses. These contradictory findings caused the group to reconvene with a core group of PCAs to determine why the scrubs were so appealing. The major reason given was that the PCA required accessible, large pockets to work efficiently. The group now had a decision to make. After considerable deliberation, and given the evidence from the available literature, the survey results, and the focused group discussions, the decision was made to have the PCA wear a navy blue polo shirt and navy cargo scrub pants.

Conclusions: The uniform choice met all the original goals. It provides a collared shirt that makes the PCA look professional and has work-friendly pants with pockets. Moreover, this uniform has helped patients recognized that the PCA is a hands-on caregiver but not a registered nurse. Although the PCAs would have liked to follow the popular scrub trend, they seem satisfied with the uniform choice. The working group will continue to assess and evaluate the uniform selection to ensure we are maintaining current standards and meeting the values and preferences of PCAs.

CHAPTER 12

Using Evidence-Based Practice to Reduce Patient Falls: Empowering Medical-Surgical Nurses

Tamara H. Murphy

I am a master's-prepared clinical nurse specialist (CNS) certified in gerontology. My studies and specialization have led me to understand the importance of scholarly work to justify the work that nurses do and to provide guidance for further practice. The challenge is in translating this research into bedside practice. This story describes the process by which a motivated nursing practice council at Penn State Hershey Medical Center (PSHMC) took ownership of the problem of patient falls on their medical-surgical unit. It also shows how crucial mentoring is to developing expertise among staff at all levels. Throughout the PSHMC Magnet journey, nursing leadership has given scholarly, evidence-based practice a high priority. I was a recently certified CNS, and the role as consultant in a project like this was new to me. The mentoring provided to me by our director of nursing research enabled me to develop my own scholarship and leadership skills throughout the process and to prepare a manuscript for publication. In turn, I found myself mentoring the nursing unit leadership and council chair to develop and use their writing and research skills. My participation at unit council meetings allowed me to strengthen my connections to the unit staff members. I was able to assist in a project that gave special attention to care of older adults, thus increasing my own visibility as a resource for expert evidence-based care of the elderly. Participation in the project also provided an opportunity for individual nursing staff to increase both their gerontological skill base and their ability to apply scholarly work to bedside care.

The Magnet journey at PSHMC created a model of shared governance that makes the staff nurse pivotal in all practice decisions. Each nursing unit at PSHMC has its own unit practice council to identify and improve practice issues. Each council sends a representative to the hospital-wide practice council, where central issues and policies are visited. The journey from a centralized nursing hierarchy to a shared governance model has challenged managers, clinical experts, and staff nurses to develop new relationships and to recognize each other's strengths and abilities in new ways. These interdependent relationships led the acute medical-surgical unit practice council to ask for my input to help them alleviate the problem of patient falls on their units.

The traditional nursing unit hierarchy places the manager as the responsible party for spearheading practice change. Under the PSHMC shared-governance model, practice and changes in practice are the domain of the staff nurse. Staff nurses are represented by peers on the governing councils. In the fall of 2006, the nurse manager for acute medicine reviewed the National Database of Nursing Quality Indicators (NDNQI) data reports with the Unit Practice Council. As is typical of many inpatient medical-surgical units that care for elderly patients, they found their unit consistently above NDNQI benchmarks for patient falls. Unit council membership, led by their council chair, engaged in the shared governance process immediately, responding to the problem of patient falls with an action plan. Together with their manager and their clinical head nurse, the council members analyzed the unit falls data and consulted the literature and the experts. They evaluated multifaceted, evidence-based interventions to determine what might have the greatest positive impact on patient care on their unit. They were prepared to use unit audit data and NDNQI quarterly reports to support the actions that they needed to take.

The council recognized that falls were particularly prevalent in persons over 65 years old on acute medical units. They looked to me, as the gerontological CNS, for help in identifying further evidence-based practices that might impact the safety of elders on their unit and lower their falls rate. They invited me to one of their meetings in the fall of 2006. As a geriatric specialist and as a CNS, I was excited to be consulted for my expertise in the care of elders and to be asked to work within the sphere of CNS practice that includes patient care, support of nursing practice, and system change.

By the time I met with the council chair, a staff nurse council member, and the nurse manager, the unit's initial falls action plan was already well under way. Their questions to me were: Is there a better screening tool? Is there a medical diagnosis or drug that might signal a need for increased surveillance? Is there any other practice change we might make to reduce our fall rate? I shared the results of my own literature review and confirmed for them that they had already implemented many of the evidence-based falls prevention measures identified in the literature. I also shared that I had been to a national gerontological meeting recently where nurses and nursing assistants from a specific hospital unit presented the results of a planned intervention to improve patient care to elders. These nurses had reeducated their nursing assistants about eldercare, solicited the nursing assistant's input for changing the bathing and activity routines of the unit, and placed the nursing assistants in charge of targeted rounds every 2 hours that addressed comfort and safety needs of patients. Their desired outcome measures were an increase in discharges to home rather than the nursing home, decreased length of stay, and increased nursing assistant satisfaction. To their delight, they also noted increased patient satisfaction, a decrease in their falls rate, and a decrease in their decubitus ulcer rate.

It was almost as if a light came on. The practice council nurses began sharing plans that they had made to institute an hourly nursing rounds program based on the work of Meade, Bursell, and Ketelson (2006). The council chair had recently disseminated their article from the *American Journal of Nursing* entitled "Effects of Nursing Rounds on Patients' Call Light Use, Satisfaction, and Safety" to the entire staff. The research findings of Meade et al. (2006) demonstrated decreased usage of call bells after instituting a special staff rounding protocol. The goal of the PSHMC nursing unit was to show that their "rounds project" would improve efficiency by reducing the number of unnecessary call bells. "That," I told them, "is going to impact your falls rate, your pressure ulcer rate, your incontinence rate, and your patient satisfaction!" Talk about synergy. We were all on the same page. This was evidence-based practice! Their research and ideas that had already been set in motion to address efficiency were going to decrease their falls rate too! This collaborative group of managers, specialists, and empowered staff nurses initially met with a shared goal to improve care for older patients by decreasing their falls rate. The group found that in this original sharing of knowledge and working together from multiple roles and viewpoints, the best practices were validated and strengthened.

Of course, the scripted, scheduled patient rounding did not occur without some obstacles. It is difficult to carry out an organized rounding routine when there are so many demands placed on staff in an acute care sitting. Maintaining hourly rounds in teams of two for each of the unit's wings required assigning them a shift ahead. It also required engaging charge nurses, RNs, LPNs, and nurses' aides in the process. Comments were encouraged from all staff members during the intervention. Benefits cited by staff nurses included anticipating the need for pain medication and the need to change an IV bag before the alarm sounded. Staff credited a better call bell response time to the fact that there were fewer calls to answer. The nurse manager said she sensed that staff felt more empowered to prioritize and organize their work. She also recognized that "efficient response to call bells has had an impact on the overall organization in terms of patient satisfaction and employee satisfaction."

The unit council members have since visited other units with fall rates above NDNQI benchmarks. They are sharing their research and data at those unit practice council meetings. One clinical head nurse shared with me, "At first they didn't like the idea, and it seemed like too much work." Then one of the council members looked at the data and said, "But you can't argue with these numbers."

The abstract describes the practice changes that were implemented and monitored by the unit practice council. It is in part an excerpt from a manuscript that we worked as a group to write. Results of the interventions indicated a decrease in the unit falls rate and an increase in patient satisfaction for the following quarter. This evidence-based practice intervention has provided positive outcomes to patient care and has validated my belief in the strength of research-based practice. Additionally, it has been a rewarding experience in developing effective work relationships within a shared governance model.

I would encourage nurses at all levels to actively engage in the change process. More and more, the influence of nursing practice can be measured by direct patient outcomes. As hospitals move toward Magnet designation, nurses are empowered with the tools to monitor and to determine their own practice. Nurses no longer need to complain and take their issues up the hierarchy, waiting for instructions or for a special "fix." In a decentralized, unit-based, shared governance model, I have witnessed staff nurses wholeheartedly embracing their practice and taking problems and salient issues to their nursing practice councils. Here they share and own the problem and the solutions. Nurses are then experiencing greater autonomy and producing improved patient care outcomes.

Falls Prevention for Elders in Acute Care: An Evidence-Based Nursing Practice Initiative

Tamara H. Murphy, MS, ACNS–BC, CCRN

Purpose: This initiative shows how staff nurses effectively used the research process to implement an evidence-based practice (falls prevention program) on their unit.

Design: The project was designed within the context of a shared governance model in which nurses at the unit level were empowered to promote quality of care by effectively implementing a falls prevention program. The group effort included reviewing unit falls data and comparing them with National Database of Nursing Quality Indicators (NDNQI) benchmarks; researching the available literature related to falls; developing an evidence-based action plan; implementing interventions; monitoring unit practices related to falls; and measuring patient outcomes.

Methods: Practice council members reviewed falls data for their unit to identify patterns and trends. Data were retrieved from a fall occurrence report. Trends on the adult medical-surgical unit resembled those reported in the literature, with 68% of patients who fell being on falls precautions; 41% of patients had altered mental status before the fall; 38% were incontinent; 26% were unable to rise from a chair before the fall; 24% had received benzodiazepines; and 18% had depression. Outcomes for patients who fell were 79% having no injury, 12% having minor injury, and 9% having moderate injury. No major injuries or deaths were reported.

The practice council also reevaluated the current institution-wide "falls precautions" policy. That policy was reviewed and updated annually according to hospital procedures. They identified additional opportunities to reduce the fall risk on their unit. They created "falls tool boxes" (U.S. Department of Veteran Affairs, 2004) that contained orange labels, magnets, wristbands, and the teaching sheets for falls prevention. These were placed on each wing in a visible area to increase the availability of these materials to staff. They recommended educating new staff and reeducating more experienced staff to ensure that all staff were using the falls precautions protocols.

Realizing the importance of the falls issues, the practice council decided to do a replication of a quasi-experimental study that evaluated the use of call lights in 14 hospitals across the United States. The unit practice council adapted the research of Meade, Bursell, and Ketelson (2006) to their own unit's special needs. They developed a plan for hourly rounds with scripted questions that addressed pain and comfort, PRN medications, toileting, and positioning. They checked for proximity of the patient's call bell, water, telephone, tissues, TV remote, bedside table, and waste can. The patient was asked if he or she needed anything else and was told that another staff member would return in an hour. The charge nurse, staff RNs, LPNs, and nursing assistants were assigned hourly rounds in pairs. Baseline data on the number of call bells were collected before implementing the practice change. Call bell numbers were tallied on a list placed outside every door. Unit leadership assisted the practice council members in monitoring compliance. Staff feedback was solicited and encouraged.

Results: Data were collected for 2 weeks after the practice change in rounds was implemented. Call rates for 2 weeks on one wing of the unit decreased from 349 to 273; the other wing's 2-week call rate decreased from 583 to 152. The rounds intervention occurred throughout Weeks 3, 4, 5, and 6. Fall rates were monitored using NDNQI quarterly reports. NDNQI unit data were compared with national benchmarks and showed that December's fall rates were below benchmark for the first time in 3 years. Patient satisfaction data for October 2006 through March 2007 showed that satisfaction with overall nursing care increased from 86% to 88%. Patient satisfaction with discharge instruction increased from 79% to 82%. Satisfaction with pain control increased from 85% to 89%. Satisfaction with information regarding patients' health condition increased from 75% to 82%.

Conclusions: The NDNQI benchmarks and the patient satisfaction data are considered to be nurse-sensitive measures. Unit leadership attributed these patient satisfaction gains to an ability to respond more quickly to fewer call bells, as well as the staff feeling more autonomy in organizing their day. Staff also noted an ability to anticipate needs for interventions, like pain medications and IV infusion changes, before the call bell was needed. Results of this unit research project show how a unit's nursing staff, empowered by a shared governance model, were able to use available benchmarking data to plan and implement practice improvements and to demonstrate positive patient outcomes. They employed the results of a literature search to identify a strategic plan and to develop interventions that might lead to a decrease in their unit falls rate. They were able to measure the success of their intervention by tracking NDNQI benchmarks and patient satisfaction data. Because there was more than one intervention (falls tool boxes, educational blitz, and scripted rounds), it is difficult to say which intervention may have had the greatest impact. Significant gains were made in both NDNQI nurse-sensitive quality indicators and in patient satisfaction scores during the time frame of the interventions and immediately afterward.

REFERENCES

Meade, C. M., Bursell, A. L., & Ketelson, L. (2006). Effects of nursing rounds on patients' call light use, satisfaction, and safety. *American Journal of Nursing, 106*(9), 58-70.

U.S. Department of Veteran Affairs. (2004). *National Center for Patient Safety 2004 Falls Toolkit.* National Center for Patient Safety. Retrieved May 30, 2007, from http://www.va.gov/ncps/SafetyTopics/fallstoolkit/index.html

Research, Recognition, and Representation: Lighting Up Interest in Evidence-Based Practice

Patricia Conway Decina and Lisa Waraksa

As staff nurses on the one and only pediatric unit in a five-hospital system in suburban Philadelphia, we have learned to advocate for our pediatric population. Fortunately for us, particularly because our enlightened hospital administrators began the Magnet journey several years ago, we believe that our voices are heard. Associated with our efforts toward Magnet recognition, our hospital system chose to adopt a unit council system of shared governance along with a clinical ladder system. The unit council structure gives us the vehicle to address, from the bedside upward, concerns about our professional practice, patient and staff satisfaction, and outcomes. The clinical ladder system promotes active continual learning and vigorous involvement on the part of nurses who are inspired to provide superior patient care and retain skilled peers as employees. The ultimate goal is ensuring optimal outcomes for members of the community who look to us to do just that for themselves and their loved ones when in our care.

Climbing the clinical ladder helps in a few particular ways. Because clinical level IV staff nurses are recognized by the hospital system as having met rigorous criteria, including performing a research project, staff nurses can easily identify them as skilled resources and mentors who value evidence-based practice. Second, because there is financial incentive associated with clinical levels III and IV, the clinical ladder system allows nurses to advance at the bedside, where patients can benefit the most. Achieving clinical level IV at our healthcare institution requires obtaining 14 points in a range of areas, including educational degrees, certifications, continuing education credits, presentations, articles and publications, memberships in professional organizations, community and organizational services, and others. In addition to points, the applicant must be interviewed by a panel of peers. Finally, applicants must pursue research. Here is where our journey begins.

As pediatric staff nurses for over 20 years, it is not an exaggeration to say that we have at least one question daily that we recruit the expertise of fellow nurses, pediatricians, case managers, or others to help answer. The response is not usually a well-defined evidence-based plan to proceed, but more often a plan carefully devised from consensus. The reason for this is that there is much research that needs to be done even about the most common nursing interventions, and there is no quick avenue to use available research at the point of care at any given moment. In addition to the inquiring minds that nurses often have, there is the strong desire to decrease the pain and suffering—not only from whatever illness or condition brought the child into the hospital but also from hospitalization itself.

When we recognized that there was a forum, the clinical ladder program, to investigate our plan of care for infants with hyperbilirubinemia, we jumped at the opportunity to change a treatment plan that we believed had associated risks that we could minimize and that was incredibly difficult for new parents to experience. The other piece of this puzzle was that our equipment was getting old and requiring more and more calls to our maintenance department for repair. We took full advantage of these circumstances. We approached the head of our nursing education department about our hope to research this topic. She referred us to our research mentor, who has been invaluable to us. With a PhD in nursing, she had taught in baccalaureate nursing programs and had served on the institutional review board in prior years. She is engaged in her own research, in assisting us and other staff nurses with research, and in fulfilling other important educational needs of the five-hospital system as well. Though her slate is full, she has advised and encouraged us. She has given us the confidence to perform our research and to present it. As an aside, it is important to mention that our institution is just going to electronic record-keeping for nursing documentation and medication administration. Within the last 2 years, nurses began using e-mail as the primary means of communication. In another year or so, physician order entry will be used. Because we use the computer for only a few limited applications, we are not computer savvy. Our peers have had more than a few laughs at our expense as they have observed our progress in this area. So, we needed to develop some very basic skills to do our research. We continue to learn as we go. One of our bigger obstacles—and accomplishments—to date is learning to create a PowerPoint presentation.

We wrote our research proposal, which was two and a half pages long. Our goal was to provide the most appropriate medical and nursing care to our children and ensure that parents can be actively involved in their care at every point during the infant's hospital stay. We briefly explained the topic of hyper-bilirubinemia, the population at risk, and the sequelae associated with ineffective treatment. We also included the American Academy of Pediatrics clinical practice guidelines and recommendations and the fact that there were Joint Commission Sentinel Event Reports issued in 2001 and 2004 related to the care of children with neonatal jaundice. We wanted our healthcare institution, which is largely focused on the adult population, to better understand that this diagnosis is an area that has received a huge amount of attention in the pediatric community over the last few years. We included our current practice, the risks inherent in it, and the difficulty associated with it for the parents. Finally, we identified that we wanted to do a comparative analysis of that practice with a different method of treatment that would be safe and effective. We stated that we would need guidance regarding sample size, ideal data collection methods, and proper analysis of the information so that we could be confident of interpreting the data correctly and truly promote the best outcome for our infants and families.

Once our proposal was accepted by the research committee, we obtained the approval of our patient care manager. The next step was to complete an exhaustive literature search on the topic. We investigated hyperbilirubinemia, the Joint Commission's recent interest and the sentinel event alerts associated with the diagnosis over the last few years, and the use of the Bilibed and other modalities for the treatment of hyperbilirubinemia. In completing this review of the literature, we were very interested in the fact that the information that the company offers in support of the product is outdated, having been published in 1997. We found few studies that reviewed the effectiveness of the Bilibed, though it was being used in a number of hospitals. We were surprised that there was little evidence to support it as a method of treatment. We believe that its popularity is due to the fact that there are few methods of delivering intensive phototherapy that allow such easy interaction between parent and infant.

We care for approximately 80–100 infants with hyperbilirubinemia each year on our unit. With that in mind, we chose a sample size of 20 infants for our study. We further defined our population to be infants in their first week of life. They were to be greater than or equal to 35 weeks gestation, without ABO incompatibility (a hemolytic process that can complicate the course of treatment), and without temperature instability.

We then had the arduous task of convincing our pediatricians of the value of the research. We could not proceed without their support. Our pediatric unit is approximately 20 beds. Our patients are fortunate to be in the care of outstanding pediatric hospitalists who are available 24 hours each day to provide, assess, evaluate, and fine-tune care. Our doctors insisted on knowing what equipment the area pediatric hospitals were using before they would consider changing our plan of care. Our next task was to survey local hospitals. Because of our location in suburban Philadelphia, there was a wide array of pediatric units and pediatric tertiary care hospitals for us to tap for information. The managers and nurse educators at these institutions were gracious enough to answer the questions on our brief survey. The Bilibed was clearly a popular alternative to the system of quadruple phototherapy that we were currently using. Some of our pediatricians were more supportive of our research than others. However, we were able to proceed because our head pediatrician was fully on board with the plan to use the Bilibed as our standard of care if the research proved it to be effective.

Next on the agenda was actually obtaining the equipment; this was not a difficult part of our project because of a grant available to us. As a result of the concern about the neurologic sequelae of untreated hyperbilirubinemia and the Joint Commission sentinel event alerts, as well as the American Academy of Pediatrics recommendations, there was a lot of interest in this topic in the world of pediatric medicine. Our hospital system made it a point to address jaundice management in the neonatal intensive care unit (NICU), in the nurseries, and on the pediatric unit. In contrast to the high profile of the condition, the cost of the equipment we were interested in using was not high. The Bilibed is such a simple piece of equipment; it is an intense blue light in a wavelength between 425 nm and 475 nm that lies underneath a soft Plexiglas pane on which the infant lies. The light penetrates the back mesh side of the suit. It is placed in a bassinet for use. The Bilibed cost $2,200. The bilibombi suits cost about $10 each, and we believed that in most cases, one or two per patient would be used. The replacement lights were inexpensive and only needed to be changed, according to manufacturer guidelines, after 1,500 hours of use. Our infant average time on the Bilibed would turn out to be less than 22 hours for a complete course of treatment.

As staff nurses who understand that there is very little time to give the comprehensive quality care to our patients given the cost of health care and the amount of time needed to complete the overwhelming amount of required documentation, we spent much time carefully considering how to go about collecting data. We were particularly interested in devising a plan for data collection that would promote buy-in of staff, that could be accomplished easily, that would not frustrate staff, and that would not leave holes that would interfere with our research. We believed that we needed to take the most simple of approaches. We chose to use our existing nursing flow sheet for our data collection. The intensity of the phototherapy light was a required value. We needed our staff nurses to be 100% compliant with recording that. In addition, we needed to know the number of hours on the Bilibed. To get that figure, the nurses zeroed the light prior to treatment and then read the number of hours that continued to tally on the Bilibed itself until the end of the treatment. We needed the total hours on the bed. Because we were fearful of someone forgetting to record, we asked for nurses to record the intensity of the light each shift. We also asked for nurses to record the number of hours on the bed each time the lights were turned off for an infant who was taken off the bed to be fed by the parents or for lab tests to be drawn. We were able to achieve all the data needed by adding these extra measures.

We were able to determine the effectiveness of the bed. We were satisfied that the Bilibed allowed parents to interact with their infant in a way that they could not with quadruple phototherapy. Unlike with the older method, in which lights were often repositioned without staff knowing, we were able to know the intensity of the light that the infant received during the course. The infant was not at risk of becoming dehydrated or losing weight because of overheating (overheating occurred with quadruple phototherapy because the intense lights would overwhelm the ability of the isolette to maintain temperature within a proper range). The risk of damage to the eyes was eliminated because the infant lies face-up on the Bilibed, unlike in quadruple phototherapy, in which the infant must wear eye patches for protection against damage to the retinas from the intense light. Parents can bond with the infant, whom they can see, touch, and hold readily when the Bilibed is used. One huge benefit of the Bilibed for staff nurses is that there is no need for hunting and gathering of the large number of pieces of equipment required for quadruple phototherapy, which caused delays in care and required a larger patient room to use.

The means for admission bilirubin, discharge bilirubin, intensity of the light, hours on the Bilibed, and length of hospital stay were determined. We currently use the Bilibed on our pediatric unit. Our research shows that the Bilibed is a safe, effective, and efficient treatment method for hyperbilirubinemia that allows us to deliver patient-centered care in a timely and cost-effective manner.

We are excited by our results. We worked many hours, and many of those hours were our own time. Our efforts have taken us on a road that we did not anticipate. Our research efforts have offered us such special and varied experiences in nursing. Because we are two of very few clinical level IV staff nurses in our health system, we are among a small number of nurses who have done research. In addition, our research was generated from needs recognized at the bedside. We are proud of that.

To elaborate on where our research has taken us, we have spoken at two research days for our health system. These events were scheduled to encourage more nursing involvement. We were invited to speak at a Sigma Theta Tau research symposium for the College of Nursing at Villanova University, where we spoke to undergraduate and graduate students, members of the faculty of Villanova, and faculty from other nearby universities who were Sigma Theta Tau members. The response there was so positive. Academic researchers offered suggestions for us about how we might proceed with our work on this topic. We benefited from this interaction with professionals who are invested in doing research to improve the health of our community. We were also encouraged by our advisor and by those spearheading the Magnet effort at our health system to present a poster at the Nursing Management Congress in Philadelphia. We wrote an abstract, which was accepted. This was yet again a different population for us, and it was interesting to speak with attendees. This was only the beginning! We were asked by our mentor to send an abstract to the Sigma Theta Tau Nursing Convention in Vienna in July 2007. We did not foresee actually presenting there. It was such thrill to actually receive the invitation and to present in an environment in which I could interact with the international nursing community. I had not traveled to Europe before, so it was a great learning experience. In a different context, our NICU nurse educator approached us several weeks ago to convey a message from an educator from a neighboring health system who had heard our Villanova presentation. She expressed that her health system was beginning the Magnet journey. She said that she was impressed by the simplicity of our approach and that she would like us to present to her nursing staff. We recently presented our research there. During that research day, it became clear to us that we have a story to tell. Our research was the only research that day that was initiated by staff nurses in response to a problem encountered on the unit. The questions we were asked showed that nurses were truly interested, though fearful. The comments were favorable, and the nurses commented that they appreciated our coming because they could identify with our motivation and our approach. The administrators and educators were interested in our story about conducting our research and about the clinical ladder system as an incentive. For our institution, our presentation to a neighboring healthcare system that will apply for Magnet designation will be used as an example of Magnet mentoring, a requirement of Magnet recognition.

Finally, our presentation was offered in abbreviated format to inspire high school students from eight area schools to be interested in health careers. At a recent career discovery day at one of our hospitals, our presentation about pediatric nursing and research gave them some exposure to the varied aspects of nursing. Our liaisons to the community have noted our work and each of our presentations in *Nursing Spectrum* and *Advance for Nurses*. Our hospital news bulletin has shown our pictures. We know that with each presentation and each article that appears about our work, our health system is gaining more exposure as a Magnet healthcare organization dedicated to research and quality. We are proud of that too.

In trying to make suggestions or comments to others who might be interested or motivated to do research, we would certainly say that it is important for staff nurses to know that limiting the scope of an initial research project, and maybe proceeding in a stepwise fashion, can be less frustrating and more successful. It is also important to recognize the limitations of the staff who will collect the data. Being realistic about your expectations of their participation is key. Chances are that you want the weekend evening nurse to be as invested as the nurse you might see each day during the week. Interacting personally with all data collectors, educating them about the research, listening to their comments, and answering their questions should be part of the plan. We believe that it is helpful to recognize that negotiating organizational constraints requires that proper supports be in place. We would have hit roadblocks that would have stopped us in our tracks if we did not have a mentor who actively educated and intervened for us. Nurses should know that the workload, even for a research project of limited scope, is heavy but rewarding. Finally, organizations would be wise to clinch their interested nurses by offering those supports and by offering a clinical ladder (or some equivalent) and financial incentives to nurses to promote practice that is evidence based and to send a message that nurses who dedicate themselves to research are highly valued.

Acknowledgment: We would like to acknowledge the expertise, guidance, and encouragement provided to us by our mentor, Dr. Ruth Mooney. Her many efforts on our behalf and her advocacy made our nursing research process interesting and enjoyable. We are grateful to our fellow nurses, pediatricians, unit secretaries, and patient care technician who helped to collect data and who supported our efforts. We would also like to thank others at Bryn Mawr Hospital, including Mary Barrett, Amy Pellig, and Claire Baldwin for their support for the Clinical Ladder Program and for the opportunity to pursue research to benefit our pediatric patients and their families. Final thanks to John Waraksa and Larry Decina for assisting in the review of this document and for their support of this project.

The Use of the Bilibed for Infants Hospitalized for Treatment of Hyperbilirubinemia

Patricia Conway Decina, BSN, RN, CPN;
and Lisa Waraksa, BS, RN, CPN

Purpose: Treatment of hyperbilirubinemia in infants using quadruple phototherapy interferes with parent–infant bonding by creating a barrier to sight, sound, and touch. The lights cause overheating and insensible fluid loss, which can prompt evaluation for sepsis in infants. The evaluation includes blood draws, lumbar puncture, and urinary catheterization and can lead to initiating IV fluid replacement and prophylactic antibiotics. Gathering the numerous pieces of equipment needed for phototherapy causes delays in treatment.

Because the infant is not enclosed in an isolette, the Bilibed allows parents easy access and fosters independence in caring for their infant. There is no heat generated by the light source, so there is no risk of unnecessary workup or treatment for fever or insensible fluid loss related to treatment.

Methodology: Twenty infants were enrolled in a study to determine effectiveness of the Bilibed. Bilirubin levels were recorded upon admission and discharge. Infants were placed on the Bilibed, and parents were instructed on its use. Irradiance, hours of phototherapy, and length of hospital stay were noted. Group means were calculated. Healthcare providers were surveyed to assess their satisfaction with the Bilibed.

Results: The means were as follows: admission bilirubin, 19.9 mg/dl; discharge bilirubin, 13.5 mg/dl; irradiance, 65.8 microwatts/cm2/nm; hours on the Bilibed, 21.9 hours; and length of hospital stay, 33.7 hours. The Bilibed is a safe, effective, efficient treatment method for hyperbilirubinemia that exemplifies patient-centered care delivered in a timely and cost-effective manner.

CHAPTER 14

Jump in with Both Feet, the Waters Get Warmer over Time!

Catherine Tieva

Nursing research, evidence-based practice, literature reviews, meta-analysis, correlations, control and experimental groups, and validity. Terms like these used to make the hair on the back of my neck stand on end. My palms would break into a sweat, and if ever I felt inadequate as a nurse, it was in the area of nursing research. I would listen to advanced practice nurses, master's-prepared nurses, and doctorate-prepared nurses discussing research and feel totally inadequate. It didn't matter that at the time, I had 16 years of experience or that I was currently working as a nurse manager. Nursing research seemed to be a foreign language. To console myself, I would say that research wasn't my cup of tea. It was too dry, too complex, and impossible to undertake in the "real world."

Over time, it became apparent to me that I could stick my head in the sand and pretend it wasn't there, but the truth was, nursing research was here to stay. I decided to get brave and test the waters. I joined the research committee at the hospital where I work. Surrounded by a number of illustrious nurses with backgrounds that were equally impressive didn't do much to bolster my confidence. I sat at the table and listened and listened, and, you guessed right, listened some more. You couldn't have called me a big contributor to the group, but rather, I like to think of myself more like a sponge. The nurses on the committee were intelligent and passionate about nursing research and about evidence-based practice (EBP). They talked about this study and that study, and which researcher would be their biggest find for the nursing research conference they were planning. I wanted to volunteer, but they seemed to have everything under control. They really didn't seem to notice little old me at the table. This was not good. Normally I am a person of action. This treading water near the banks of the research river would never do. I decided I would have to start swimming.

It just so happened that about this time, the organization I work for was offering 16 individuals from various departments in the hospital the opportunity to learn basic skills to lead an EBP project of their own. Dr. Marita Titler,

Laura Cullen, and Hope Barton from the University of Iowa Hospitals and Clinics were coming to present a 3-day educational session complete with an EBP toolkit that would help us find our way down the "river of EBP."

I was excited. Staff members who were interested in participating in this educational opportunity were required to fill out an application. Applicants needed to give an overview of their background and indicate what type of project they would carry out if given an opportunity. That is where I met my first roadblock. Applicants were required to have a minimum of a BSN. I only had an associate degree in nursing (ADN).

As I said earlier, I am a person of action. Undaunted, I submitted my application. I wanted to learn, and if I didn't apply, I would not have any chance to participate. Several weeks later, I received news that I had been selected as one of the 16 nurses in the organization to participate in the educational sessions. I was ecstatic and prepared to attempt to paddle down the river of EBP once again. That said, you may be wondering what project I decided to undertake. I work on an oncology unit. Fatigue is a problem that is experienced by nearly all cancer patients undergoing treatment. According to the Oncology Nursing Society (ONS), fatigue is the least assessed, educated about, and addressed side effect of cancer overall. I thought that this would make an excellent project. It could be carried out not only on the inpatient unit but in the outpatient, radiation oncology, chemo infusion, home care, and outreach settings as well.

Nervous, hesitant, and armed with a basic course on EBP, I remained determined, and I set out to undertake my first official EBP project. I have to admit that the waters weren't always smooth, and I needed a life preserver of encouragement along the way, but I did it! I learned by trial and error. I am happy to report that the cancer fatigue project has been implemented. I have more confidence, and in fact, I have undertaken several other projects using research to guide the way.

Each time, it gets a little bit easier. For a person who didn't have a clue where to begin several years ago, I can say without hesitation that undertaking EBP projects is not only fun but also the right thing to do for our patients and their families. There is literature out there that can guide you along the way. If you have never attempted an EBP project, my suggestion is, "Come on in, the water is fine!"

Acknowledgment: The author would like to recognize the expertise of Roxanne Wilson, Internal Medicine Care Center director at St. Cloud, and Sandy Johnson, oncology clinical nurse specialist, for the guidance, patience, and expertise they provided to me as a novice utilizing evidence-based knowledge in my practice.

Implementation of a Formal Process to Provide Assessment, Education, and Interventions for Cancer-Related Fatigue Utilizing EBP

Catherine Tieva, BA, RN, OCN

Purpose: The Oncology Nursing Society (ONS) identified a cluster of side effects experienced by nearly all cancer patients undergoing treatment. Cancer-related fatigue (CRF) is the most prevalent side effect of cancer treatment. It is also the least addressed. CRF is a distressing, persistent, subjective sense of tiredness or exhaustion related to cancer or cancer treatment that is not proportional to recent activity and interferes with usual functioning. Education is an important part of treatment. By understanding fatigue, patients can cope better as well as reduce distress.

A multidisciplinary team comprising healthcare professionals from the inpatient oncology unit, the outpatient cancer center, radiation oncology, home care services, and outreach clinics worked together to become clinical experts on the subject of CRF. The goal was to improve care delivered to the oncology patient population by implementing a formal process to provide assessment, education, and interventions for CRF utilizing evidence-based practice.

Design: Synthesis of the Evidence/Levels of Evidence: This was accomplished by synthesizing information available in both literature and guidelines. The National Commission on Cancer (2005) developed *Guidelines for the Management of Fatigue*, which summarized standards of care for fatigue assessment and management based on an extensive synthesis of evidence (Level A). By familiarizing themselves with the evidence, the team was able to develop methods to assist caregivers in supporting this particular patient population. Further literature reviews were required when guidelines were updated several times over the course of this project and when the FDA released a change in recommended treatment.

Proposed Change in Practice: Use, adapt, and develop formal assessment tools based on available evidence. Develop patient and staff education materials appropriate for the level of patient fatigue assessed.

Methods: Evaluation/Outcome Measures Premeasure: Measurements were taken of nursing and provider assessment of, interventions for, and patient education on, fatigue. This was accomplished through staff knowledge surveys and performing retrospective baseline chart audits. Results showed that providers possessed a fair amount of baseline knowledge on the subject of CRF, but limited documentation of assessment, education, or interventions provided to patients was being done.

Implementation Strategies: The teams agreed on a project theme and logo. A baseline assessment tool was adopted from the ONS. Using available research, a subgroup developed a comprehensive fatigue assessment tool. Educators developed a patient education sheet, and the team's oncology clinical nurse specialist assisted with designing a standard of care, policy, and standing orders for project use. Piloted implementation began in the inpatient setting in February 2007, which correlated with the hospital's electronic medical record system going live. Outpatient chemo infusion and radiation went live in April 2007. Outreach and home care are not yet up and running.

Results: Evaluation/Outcome Measures Postimplementation: Postimplementation audit results showed nursing improvements in all areas. Nursing documentation increased by 32%, documented education increased by 33%, and documented management strategies improved by 32% when measured in August 2007.

Next Steps: Sustain the gains already made. Facilitate further process improvements through postimplementation focus groups with participation by staff and patients. Evaluate findings, review literature on a regular basis, and fine-tune current project work.

Conclusions: Initial prospective chart audits indicate that steps taken to address fatigue in the oncology patient population have resulted in improvements in documented assessments, interventions, and education by nurses. There remains a need to continue to measure and report progress through the organization's performance improvement system. It appears feasible to explore opportunities to carry out this work in other patient populations in the future.

Say "Yes!" to Research

Sheree O'Neil

I have always respected research findings as an integral part of the professional nurse's practice and admired those knowledgeable and skilled enough to pursue that specialty. However, I was never quite sure what the day-to-day activities of the nurse researcher would be, whom she would be responsible to, and where she might practice. The sheer management of a large research project seemed overwhelming, and the potential for error intimidating. The concept was, for me, basically an unknown variable, a black hole. Besides, the focus of my career had always been on the patient and his or her clinical issues. Nursing research seemed far removed from my realm—pretty ivory tower stuff. However, my view changed several years ago when our institution began its pursuit of Magnet status, and I was fortunate to be asked to participate as a Magnet Champion. This assignment placed me on several committees and in meetings where I began to hear about the increased emphasis on evidence-based practice. I became aware of the research projects already under way in our hospital and witnessed the excitement they generated. I also saw the commitment and support dedicated to them by senior management.

As the population of our county grew, so did the inpatient unit on which I have worked for many years. Additional policies and procedures needed to be written, but the lack of research on which to base these new protocols delayed and confused the process. With more and more nurses asking about the foundations of their everyday practices, the need for more nursing research became more and more pressing in my immediate practice. I knew that the Inova Loudoun Hospital offered a 2-day clinical research course and a nursing research internship program to instruct and support nurses in their research. These programs were more evidence to me that Inova Loudoun Hospital was serious about supporting their staff nurses' development along the practice continuum toward autonomy and accountability. These forces worked to lessen my resistance to the idea of participation in a research project.

My research question developed during a conversation with another nurse and our chief nursing officer (CNO) while attending a Magnet conference. At dinner, our CNO expressed her concern about the continued violation of policy and procedure despite the recent implementation of numerous safety efforts and a very large effort to change the safety culture. Even an increased awareness of the consequences of a safety violation had not reduced the numbers of incidents. We wondered together, "Why are the staff continuing to make mistakes despite the added focus on error prevention?" We agreed that we needed to determine the factors that contributed to errors in patient care not only to protect our patients from harm but also to protect our nurses from a possible career-ending episode. My coworker and I were asked by our CNO to research the possible explanations for the continued safety violations. Because of the influences that lessened our resistance to the idea of participation in research and an urgency to protect our patients and staff, when our CNO asked us to look into these causes, we were able to say "Yes" to research.

My participation, first as a Magnet Champion and now as a nurse research intern, has been a time of exponential growth for my nursing practice, and I am truly grateful for the experience. Through this internship, I have been given the opportunity to continue on my professional journey from novice practitioner toward expert nurse. Many areas of my professional practice have matured. This position encouraged improvement in computer and library skills and an enhanced understanding of the research process. Insight into the patient safety body of knowledge, my study topic, was gained and is now incorporated into my patient side practice. An awareness and appreciation of the safety movement in health care has become of special importance to me, and I have made a personal commitment to help nurses develop strategies to reduce errors.

As I distributed and gathered surveys, I had the opportunity to speak with staff about the research opportunities at Inova Loudoun and encourage them to bring their questions to the research table. Their passion for providing safe patient care was evident. As I in-serviced managers on the completion of the Tier II survey, their eagerness to integrate research findings into their practice and help their staff practice safely made me very proud to be a member of the Inova Loudoun family.

My courage to undertake a research project was bolstered by the partnership with a coworker in the early phases of the project. We undertook the process together and collaborated on the review of the literature and study design. A dedicated person to problem-solve with in the early stages of the process saves time lost to uncertainty. Ultimately, one researcher must assume responsibility for the written documents, but I would recommend to any first-time researcher that he or she bring a friend along. The personal relationship that grows from the working relationship is an added bonus.

The journey toward Magnet status at Inova Loudoun Hospital, and for me as well, was a sincere effort toward achieving excellent patient care through the professional development of its staff. In Magnet circles, the cliché "It's about the journey" is well known. In my case, I was fortunate to be along for the ride.

Acknowledgment: Throughout the research process, I enjoyed terrific mentorship by our director of nursing research, Karen Gabel Speroni, PhD, RN. Her patience, guidance, and valuable experience were generously given to me as she shared her passion for research. I was frequently impressed by the interest and financial commitment shown by Inova Loudoun Hospital's senior leadership and the cooperation of our quality department. Their influence and confidence created a nurturing environment in which I was able to sharpen my critical thinking skills and practice in a more purposeful, systematic, and outcome-driven manner.

A Two-Tier Study of Direct Care Providers Assessing the Effectiveness of the Red Rule Education Project and Precipitating Factors Surrounding Red Rule Violations

Sheree O'Neil, MSN, RN;
Gina Harrison, BS, RN; Karen Gabel Speroni, PhD, RN;
and Marlon G. Daniel, MPH, MHA

The study was completed in 2007 at Inova Loudoun Hospital, a suburban hospital with 155 beds.

Background: In 2002, "The Joint Commission on the Accreditation of Healthcare Organizations (JCAHO) instituted new patient safety initiatives to reduce patient medical errors in the hospital setting" (O'Neill et al., 2004, p. 488). National patient safety goals were established. The first safety goal was "to improve the accuracy of patient identification using at least two patient identifiers, neither to be the patient's room number whenever taking blood samples or administering medications or blood products" (JCAHO, 2004, p.1). The Inova Hospitals implemented a Red Rule Policy and adopted this patient safety goal as their number one Red Rule. A second Red Rule was established, stating that "I will confirm the correct action or procedure before I begin" (Performance Improvement International, [PII,] 2005, p. 59). These two Red Rules were defined by Inova "as the critical requirements for safety associated with an activity or procedure on a patient that has been known to compromise patient safety" or "what we must do 100% of the time" (PII, 2005, p. 57). All direct care providers were required to complete the mandatory Red Rules Education Project, which included instruction on an error prevention technique that requires the provider to "Stop, Think, Act, and Review, or S.T.A.R." (PII, 2005, p. 68).

Purpose: The purpose of the first tier of the study is to quantify the Inova Loudoun Hospital (ILH) direct care provider's knowledge of the information taught in the Red Rule Education Project. Understanding the effectiveness of the education project will dictate the creation or modification of strategies to improve the safety culture. Because nursing and quality research have identified harmful forces that influence safe behaviors in the workplace, it is important to determine which forces continue to operate in the departments of ILH. The purpose of the second tier of the study is to determine the precipitating circumstances surrounding the occurrence of Red Rule violations. This information is essential to understanding the etiology of these events and will ideally contribute to the design of future counseling and educational efforts. As ILH implements safety initiatives to improve the safety culture at Inova Loudoun, the level of information must become increasingly specific to create strategies to prevent these safety events from occurring.

Design: Tier I was an anonymous, prospective survey research study that assessed ILH direct care providers' (e.g., RNs, LPNs, patient care technicians [PCTs], pharmacists, and pharmacy technicians) knowledge of the Red Rule Education Program. This study was conducted over a 2-month period in 2007. Tier II is an anonymous, prospective research study that surveys Red Rule violators and the precipitating circumstances surrounding the incident. It is ongoing.

Methods: During the Red Rule Awareness component of the study, 128 direct care providers (e.g., RNs, LPNs, PCTs, pharmacists, and pharmacy technicians) were surveyed during unit staff meetings and proctored by the nurse investigator. These employees were asked to take approximately 15 minutes to complete the survey at that moment and place it in the envelope provided by the proctor. A total of 118 surveys were distributed and 128 were completed, producing a 92% response rate.

Results: Univariate and bivariate analysis were performed for each Red Rule Definition. Chi-square and Fisher's Exact Test were used where appropriate. SAS (version 9.1.3; SAS Institute Inc., Cary, NC) was used to perform data management and statistical analysis.

Fewer than half (42%) of the respondents correctly identified Red Rule Definition 1, 18% were partially correct, and 39% were incorrect. Three (25%) of the 12 departments participating achieved a 50% or greater correct response rate. For Red Rule Definition 2, 9% of the sample gave correct responses, 3% gave partially correct responses, and 87% gave incorrect responses. Only one department achieved a 50% correct response rate. Only 9% of direct care providers were able to correctly identify the S.T.A.R. definition, and 28% were partially correct. A significant association between job title and correct Red Rule 1 responses was found ($p = 0.0079$). The RN correct response rate was 42%, and pharmacists received the highest rate of 60% correct for Red Rule 1. Part-time RNs received the highest percentage (50%) of correct responses for

Red Rule 1, with part-time staff receiving 47% and full-time staff receiving 41%. Float pool and agency staff received the lowest rates (0% each). Education and increased staffing were identified by providers as the top two safety efforts necessary to decrease the violation rate (21% each). Seventy-three percent of staff identified a safety effort that they would like to see implemented.

Conclusions: From an evidence-based practice viewpoint, study results conclude that the Red Rule Education Project should be enhanced and reinforced in such a manner that direct care providers can correctly define the Red Rules and S.T.A.R. error prevention technique.

REFERENCES

The Joint Commission. (2004). *2004 National Patient Safety Goals.* Retrieved November 14, 2008, from http://www.jointcommission.org/GeneralPublic/NPSG/04_gp_npsg.htm

O'Neill, K., Bradley, D., Hawkins, H., Holleran, R., Burke, P., & Hohenhaus, S., et al. (2004). Patient misidentification in a pediatric emergency department: Patient safety and legal perspectives. *Pediatric Emergency Care, 20*(7), 487–492.

Performance Improvement International. (2005). Error prevention for Inova health system employees. *Inova Health Systems Leadership Safety Training,* 57–59.

Rogers, A. E., Hwant, W. T., Scott, L. D., Aiken, L. H., & Dinges, D. F. (2004). The working hours of hospital staff nurses and patient safety. *Health Affairs, 23*(4), 202–212.

CHAPTER 16

The Rigors of Research

Laurel Barbour

Eight years ago, I accepted a new oncology advanced practice nurse role, moving from surgical oncology to medical oncology. Prior to this advanced practice nursing position, I had not conducted an entire research study. I felt inadequate to perform and bring to fruition any research study. In the past, I experienced being given wrong or inadequate information and a lack of support to perform nursing research studies. As I began to learn about the intensive therapies to treat malignant melanoma, my interest in symptom management was piqued. The physician, pharmacist, and I shared a distaste for meperidine, the standard of care, for Interleukin-2 induced rigors. We began to talk about the lack of evidence for meperidine, or any other narcotic, in the treatment of rigors. It was through the encouragement of this multidisciplinary group that I moved forward as principal investigator on the research study, titled "Placebo-Controlled, Double-Blind Trial of Intravenous Morphine Sulfate for the Treatment of Rigors."

The initial plan was slow to develop as we talked about how to conduct the trial. Staff nurses and resident physicians were brought in as part of the workgroup to provide them with exposure to the research process. I found it very important to use all the expertise and talents of each member of the multidisciplinary research group.

Since the trial, I have felt a huge sense of accomplishment. During the trial, our hospital went through the Magnet application and review. There were many accolades from nursing administration for my study. A scientific poster was made and presented in five research forums. I feel humbled, because everything was not smooth sailing; I had to rewrite the institutional review board application, I discovered that there was not an exact time at which the nurse needed to administer the medication, and we did not achieve statistical significance.

I would caution nurses not to work alone in conducting nursing research. Providing clinical care and performing nursing research take much longer than most investigators estimate. Surround yourself with excellent mentors, a doctoral-prepared nurse, a statistician, and a supportive administrator. Always double-check that as you are performing the study, you are doing the correct things statistically and ethically. Never discard any study or data-related information.

Although nursing research can be very arduous, the rewards of knowing that in some way I have helped advance nursing practice and improved the care of my patients is well worth the "rigor."

Acknowledgment: I wish to thank Dr. Jon Richards for his clinical research leadership in accomplishing this project to improve symptom management and to the oncology nursing staff at Advocate Lutheran General Hospital who carried out the research with enthusiasm.

Evidence for Biologic Therapy Rigor Control: Placebo-Controlled Trial of Intravenous Morphine

Laurel Barbour, RN, APN;
Jane Kosirog-Glowacki, PharmD, BCPS; Jon Richards, MD, PhD;
Sowjanya Reganti, MD; Jane Frugo-Denten, MSN, RN, CNA-BC;
and Paula Goff, BSN, RN, OCN

Purpose: Rigors are an unpleasant side effect experienced by patients receiving Interleukin-2 (IL2). Patients with melanoma who receive IL2 may experience serious side effects (capillary leak syndrome, renal insufficiency). The ideal rigor treatment would be effective, have minimal toxicity, and avoid overlapping IL2 toxicity.

Design: We performed a randomized double-blind trial in 38 patients receiving IL2 to determine whether morphine is effective for treatment of IL2-induced rigors.

Methods: Adult opioid naive patients received morphine 5 mg, or placebo IV push, at the first rigor from IL2. Response was assessed 5 minutes after first study dose. If rigors did not resolve after the initial 5 minutes, a second dose of the study drug was administered (maximum 2 doses, study complete after 10 minutes). If rigors continued after the second dose or recurred within 10 minutes of resolution, further management was at the physician's discretion.

Results: The primary outcome was resolution of rigors. Data (resolution, time to resolution, administration times, vital signs, pulse oximetry, adverse effects) were collected. Of 38 patients enrolled, 15 were excluded (1 received opioids, 7—no rigors, 7—treatment interval > 10 minutes). Of 23 evaluable patients, 14 received morphine, and 9 received placebo. Rigor resolution was 92.9% in morphine and 66.7% in placebo groups ($p = .264$).

CHAPTER 17

Taking a Leap into Research

Sylvia M. Belizario

I thought about going into research during my first university forestry laboratory assignment. I went up the mountain with my classmates to collect various types of leaves with different shapes, textures, and colors, identify their scientific names, and then group them according to their classification. But after I switched to nursing, I didn't think about research again until I was in graduate school. Three years later, I took a few lectures on nursing research and had several weeks of clinical experiences at the National Institutes of Health to complete my neuroscience nursing certificate program. My interest in research was rekindled, but only for a very short time; I was afraid to do it on my own then. Soon after, I had a family crisis and obligations to fulfill, so my interest in research stayed dormant until I got involved in a benchmarking project with a neurologist, after which I assisted in mentoring two neurology residents who were doing research studies. One of the residents used the benchmarking study that I had done with the neurologist to conduct his research, and he presented it at the National Medical Association conference. After this, I did not have the opportunity to get involved in research for a number of years until I came to Georgetown University Hospital as a temporary part-time nurse at the Brain & Spine Acute Care unit.

After completing my assignment and at least two unit-based performance projects—namely, documentation of medication omissions and pain reassessment—my nurse manager asked me to do a research study on the BladderScan with a colleague who was a nurse educator in order to reduce urinary tract infections in the Brain & Spine Acute Care unit. I had mixed feelings about doing a research study because I had not been involved in research for a long time and never did it on my own. I was afraid that I would not be good at it, and I was unsure about how much time would be required to complete it. I talked to a friend who challenged me. She told me that research follows the scientific method, which is a problem-solving process, and because I had done a number of performance improvement projects that involved problem solving and had some training, I should be able to do a research study. It was a very encouraging conversation, and I thought, "She's right! I will do it!" In fact, I already started developing a sort of map in my head on how to go about this

101

research study. A few days later, I wavered because I felt that even if I could do it, I wasn't that good. This vacillation of thoughts and feelings went on so many times that I just decided not to think about it—until one day when the manager told me that she had set up a meeting with someone at the General Clinical Research Center and that I must be there. Before I could tell the nurse manager about my mixed feelings and preference to just do a PI project, she told me that I could do this research study because I was already good at doing PI projects—almost the same thing that my friend had told me. When I went to the meeting, I knew that there was no backing out, and I just took the plunge! I found that much of the discussion and a number of the suggestions were in line with my thoughts, and that really encouraged me. I realized that even after being inactive for a number of years, I was not too far behind after all. This meeting took out a chunk of my fears and insecurities, and I went on to do the research study with my colleague.

When I looked into the practice of the nursing staff regarding the use of urinary catheters, I learned that they discontinued using urinary catheters on their patients—specifically, postoperative patients—as soon as possible, which was a good thing. However, the nursing staff reinserted the catheters when patients did not void within 4 hours of discontinuing the catheter, or after patients' first voiding to check postvoid residuals. Every nursing staff member I talked to informed me unequivocally that this had always been the practice. So what about the fact that frequent catheterizations increase the risk that patients will develop urinary tract infections? The number of urinary tract infections in the unit had reached an undesirable rate as benchmarked against the National Nosocomial Infection Surveillance (NNIS) rate of 7.8%. Would we be successful in stopping this nursing staff practice and changing it to using a noninvasive device such as the BladderScan?

After doing this research study, I was elated to see that the nursing staff had continued to use the BladderScan and had made it a part of their practice in the unit. A year after the study, the neurosurgery team requested a change in the protocol: If the patient's postvoid residual is high based on the Bladder-Scan, the nurse should reinsert a urinary catheter and inform the physician rather than inform the physician first and then obtain an order for recatheterization. The financial benefits resulting from this study were used to justify the purchase of a BladderScan for the surgical floor where the coinvestigator of this study works. Three years after the completion of the study, all the neuroscience nurses are very efficient in the use of the BladderScan.

Everybody starts his or her research journey from different points. For instance, one nurse may be good with numbers; another nurse may have earned her first degree in mathematics and so is even better with numbers; and yet another person may be an expert, as in a biostatistician. On the other hand, one can start without knowing anything about statistics and learn it step by step. In any case, I would encourage nurses who want to do research for the first time to attend any nursing research classes offered by their employer and start seeking out resources, such as the library, the Internet, computers, nurses, and so on. Look for a mentor and also look for a partner who is interested in doing research as well—one who is willing to learn and risk making mistakes with you, one who will share both the fun and seriousness of doing a study, and one who will share ownership of, and responsibility for, the outcome of the study. Once you have done a study, don't wait too long to get involved in another one. The longer you wait, the harder it becomes to start again. As they say, practice makes perfect; but I say, practice builds up courage, too.

Integrating the BladderScan into Standard Nursing Practice of Bladder Volume Assessments to Reduce the Frequency of Intermittent Catheterizations in Hospitalized Patients

Sylvia M. Belizario, BSN, MEd, CNRN

There are different types of hospital-acquired infections, and urinary tract infection (UTI) is just one of them; however, it is the most common one, constituting 40% of all hospital-acquired infections, and 80% of these are due to urinary catheterization or use of indwelling urinary catheters. Numerous studies have been performed that proved the effectiveness of the BladderScan in reducing UTIs and overall care costs in hospitalized patients, such as those published by Moore and Edwards (1997), Philips (2000), and Trzepacz and Fitzgerald (2002).

Purpose: This study was conducted to obtain data that will show that the use of the BladderScan can be integrated into standard nursing practice in the neuroscience unit at Georgetown University Hospital. In so doing, the frequency of intermittent and unnecessary catheterizations will be reduced.

Design: This study was designed as a descriptive study that used nonrandomized sampling of neuroscience patients who consented to participate in the study. The following protocol was developed, and all the professional staff in the unit received the same training on it and on the use of the BladderScan.

A data collection tool was developed that included the date and time that the indwelling urinary catheter was discontinued; the date, time, and bladder volume when the patient was scanned; the date, time, and reason for reinsertion of the urinary catheter; and urine output. A column for comments was also included in the tool. The staff enter data on the data collection tool as soon as the bladder scan is done on each patient. If the indwelling urinary catheter is reinserted and then discontinued again, another entry is made after

Figure 17-1   BladderScan Protocol: Brain & Spine Acute Care Unit

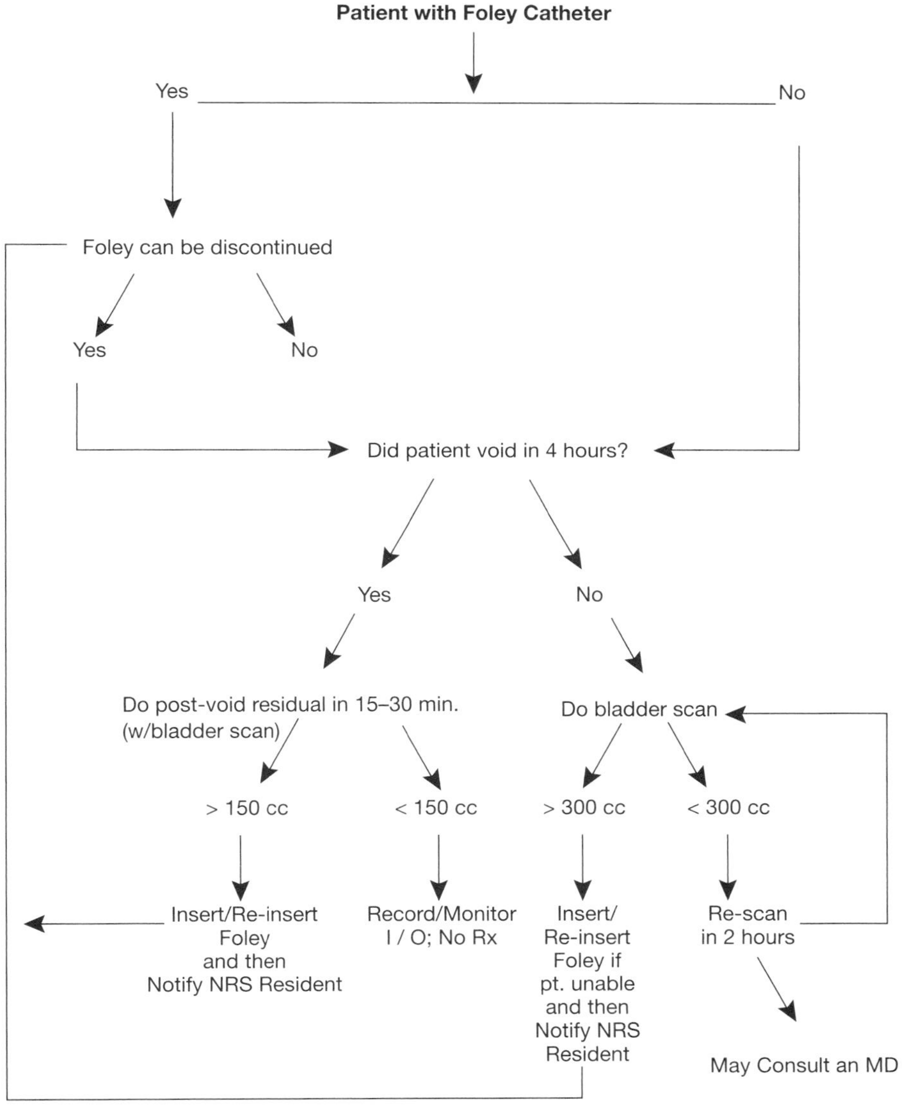

the bladder scan is done. In addition, the staff were to use a preprinted progress note for each patient on whom the BladderScan was used. The protocol, which was in the form of an algorithm, was placed in the same binder as the data collection tool and the preprinted progress notes. The study was to be completed at the end of 6 months, or when a total of 300 participants was reached.

Methods: The various methods used to gather data for this study included seeking permission from patients who were considered as potential subjects; documentation of findings on the data collection tool; documentation of the procedure in the preprinted progress notes, which should be filed in the patient's medical record; observation of staff while doing a bladder scan or inserting an indwelling urinary catheter; and chart reviews.

Results: A total of 140 bladder scans were performed on 94 neuroscience patients during the study from November 18, 2003, to June 20, 2004. Out of these 140 bladder scans, 61.4% followed the bladder scan protocol, and 38.6% deviated from it. The deviations were patient-related (27.8%) when patients were off the unit when they voided or when the patients voided without letting the nurse know about it; staff-related (63%) when the protocol was not followed (including doctors and nurses); and undetermined (9.2%) because of lack of documentation. Out of the 94 patients who consented to the study, 25 required recatheterizations. The majority of them (17) required one recatheterization before their bladders were determined to be functioning normally, and 7 of the patients required two to three reinsertions of the urinary catheter. Six patients were discharged with urinary drainage catheters because of urinary retention.

There was a daily average of 2–3 patients admitted to the neuroscience unit with urinary catheters, mostly postoperative spine patients; when a catheter was inserted, it took the staff an average of 15–20 minutes to do it, and 5–10 minutes to do a bladder scan.

Based on the number of catheterization kits saved during the study because of the use of the BladderScan instead of the kits, the unit saved about $1,800. By using the BladderScan Bladder Volume Instrument Cost Justification from Diagnostic Ultrasound, a total average annual savings of $20,000–$26,000 was projected for the Brain & Spine Acute Care unit.

Immediately after the completion of the study, the nursing staff continued to use the BladderScan, and when the neuroscience unit expanded into three units, the bladder scanner was shared among them. The clinical service manager of the general surgery unit where the coinvestigator of this study worked used the results and outcomes of this study to justify a request for a bladder scanner. After a year, the neurosurgery residents requested that the BladderScan protocol be changed to reflect that the nursing staff, without obtaining an order from them, can reinsert an indwelling urinary catheter once the patient has a postvoid residual of >150 cc or a bladder volume of 300 cc within 4 hours of the discontinuation of the urinary catheter. The nursing staff will only notify residents of a patient failing the voiding trial so that the discontinuation of the indwelling urinary catheter can be reordered the following day or the next. A policy and procedure was developed, presented to, and approved by the practice council in 2005.

Conclusion: This study showed that using the BladderScan as part of the standard practice of the staff reduced the number of unnecessary catheterizations that had been done on adult neuroscience patients to check bladder volumes; it showed that the nurses' time checking bladder volumes was shorter, and the procedure was easy, thus changing the practice of the nursing staff.

REFERENCES

Moore, D. A., & Edwards, K. (1997). Using a portable bladder scan to reduce the incidence of nosocomial urinary tract infections. *MedSurg Nursing, 6*(1), 39–43.

Phillips, J. K. (2000). Integrating bladder ultrasound: Into a urinary tract infection-reduction project. *American Journal of Nursing Supplement, 100*(Suppl. 3), 3–14.

Trzepacz, E., & Fitzgerald, J. (2002). The scan that saves. *Advance for Nurses, 2*(13), 14–16.

CHAPTER 18

You Can Teach an Old Nurse New Tricks!

Cindy Ward

After 23 years as a diploma RN graduate, I enrolled in an RN-to-MSN program at the University of Southern Indiana (USI). Over the years, I had completed a B.A. and an M.S. in health administration, but didn't feel satisfied because my degrees were not in nursing. I have remained at the bedside on a surgical unit throughout my career. I was aware of the existence of nursing research and evidence-based practice but didn't really feel that research was something that I could participate in. Although there were several topics that I had questions about and wanted to investigate, I thought that research was something that only nurses with advanced degrees were able to do.

When I enrolled in the RN-to-MSN program, I knew that research was part of the curriculum. I approached the research courses with some trepidation; however, I realized that I was there to learn and that the purpose of the courses was to begin my education about nursing research. The research class included MSN students from the various specialty tracks at USI, which included clinical nurse specialist, family nurse practitioner, acute care nurse practitioner, nursing education, and nursing leadership tracks. The professor provided us with a choice of topics of interest to the various specialties. I have long been a supporter of medical-surgical nursing as a specialty and am an active member of the Academy of Medical-Surgical Nurses, so I was pleased to see the topic "comparison of the job satisfaction of experienced medical-surgical and critical care nurses." I was excited about the topic and began to feel that maybe the class, and research in general, could be enjoyable.

The class proceeded in a step-by-step manner and led us through the various stages of setting up and conducting a research project, such as the literature review, identification of the problem, development of the hypothesis, and completion of the institutional review board application, all the way through the design and implementation of the study. My research partner was a critical care nurse, and we were both certain that our research would support our hypothesis that critical care nurses would report higher levels of job satisfaction than medical-surgical nurses. I was pleasantly surprised when our study found that there was no significant difference in the levels of job satisfaction between the two groups!

Now, my belief is that all nurses have the potential to identify research problems and participate in research to investigate their questions. I think that problems identified by bedside nurses are of great interest and relevance to other bedside nurses, and I am interested in developing and participating in more research projects. My advice to other nurses to help overcome their fears of research is to jump in and get involved in a research project, or take a research class. Either one will help the nurse learn the steps involved. Once each step is taken separately, research doesn't seem to be such a daunting task.

Acknowledgment: I would like to thank Dr. Barbara Davis and Dr. Martha Sparks at the University of Southern Indiana for their guidance through the research project. I also would like to thank my colleagues at Centra Health who have supported me as I obtained my MSN. In particular, I would like to thank Dr. Cindy Goodrich for her mentorship in research and writing, and Judy Plourde for her encouragement and support.

Comparison of the Job Satisfaction of Experienced Medical-Surgical and Critical Care Nurses

Cindy Ward, MS, RNC, CMSRN; and Sarah Shultz, MSN, RN

Data collection occurred over a 2-week period, from January 2006 to February 2006.

Purpose/Aims: To test the hypothesis that experienced (> 5 years) critical care nurses will express higher levels of job satisfaction than experienced (> 5 years) medical-surgical nurses.

Design: The study was based on Imogene King's Theory of Goal Attainment for creating improved job satisfaction for professional nurses. The instrument used was Atwood and Hinshaw's Job Satisfaction Scale (1984), along with five items from Slavitt et al.'s (1978) Index of Work Satisfaction.

Methods: The instrument and a self-addressed stamped envelope were placed in the mailboxes of all nurses who met criteria for inclusion in the study. A follow-up postcard was distributed 2 weeks later to maximize response rate.

Results: A total of 154 surveys were sent to the subjects. There were 79 valid responses (51%): 41 (51.9%) from medical-surgical nurses and 38 (48.1%) from critical care nurses. The mean number of years of experience was 19.

The Cronbach's alpha for the combined scales was acceptable at .720.

An independent t test was performed on each of the following variables: quality of care, $t(77) = -1.620$, $p = .109$; enjoyment, $t(77) = -.664$, $p = .509$; time to do one's job, $t(77) = -.670$, $p = .505$; and task requirement, $t(77) = -1.713$, $p = .091$.

No significant difference was found in the level of job satisfaction between the medical-surgical nurses and the critical care nurses.

Conclusions/Recommendations: Medical-surgical and critical care nurses in the study did not have significantly different levels of job satisfaction. No direct change in practice is warranted because of the small sample size. The recommendation is to explore a larger sample size at a variety of types of hospitals using a different type of sampling.

CHAPTER 19

Initiating a Research Project: From Mentee to Mentor

Mary Ann Francisco

I never thought I would be conducting nursing research. I had only participated in a group research project in graduate school, which was more than 25 years ago. I thought research was for academicians and nurses working with physicians in collaborative practice. I am a clinical nurse specialist certified in gerontology and work in an acute care setting. I participated in interdisciplinary quality assurance projects related to diabetes management of inpatients. Our goals were to standardize care of patients, identify target goals, and develop standardized order sets. Substantial work was completed, but when it came time to implement the project, key physician groups had conflicting opinions.

Another interdisciplinary group formed and developed goals for implementing tight glycemic control for critical care patients. These efforts were led by a new physician, so I had high expectations that we would be collectively working to implement changes that would lead to better patient outcomes. Because of my years of experience caring for patients with diabetes, my interest in exploring the cause of the increasing numbers of inpatients who were hyperglycemic, and my previous work with the quality assurance projects, I was inspired to develop a research project surrounding nursing knowledge of inpatient diabetes management. But how to go about implementing a research project?

I was nervous; I needed to find a physician who would be the principal investigator of the project. I had to review how to conduct a literature review, develop a research proposal and an abstract, complete the required forms, and submit the proposal to the hospital's institutional review board (IRB). At this time, I was fortunate to have the support of a physician who had just joined our institution and was attempting to implement standardized orders for inpatients with hyperglycemia. Additionally, I shared the idea of a research project with my unit director and received the support of the newly hired nurse researcher for the institution.

I was encouraged to expand in my role as a clinical nurse specialist, partnering with staff nurses to develop more widespread evidence-based quality initiatives that would impact large patient populations and have impact on the organization as a whole. At the time, I was ready to submit the research protocol to the IRB while precepting a staff nurse in graduate school who was completing her final coursework in the clinical nurse specialist program. She was very interested in my research project, so together we incorporated components of the research process into her objectives for her graduate work. It was a very successful relationship as I took on the role of being a mentor.

PROBLEM THAT LED ME TO CONDUCT THE STUDY

As mentioned, I was interested in the reason that so many inpatients were hyperglycemic and what nurses could do to improve their outcomes while they were hospitalized and help prevent readmission. I reviewed the American Diabetes Association standards, conducted an extensive literature review, and realized that patient outcomes and length of stay could be greatly impacted just by keeping patients' blood sugars under control. Newer treatment standards, newer insulins, and newer research findings were available for integration into nursing practice. Staff nurses needed this information to successfully care for patients, so I collaborated with the outpatient certified diabetes educator to develop some educational sessions for the medical-surgical nurses throughout the institution.

These sessions were the beginning of a program on diabetes education for staff, but I still considered whether the content of the education was appropriate and up to date. I began to ponder what further content needed to be developed. What was the current knowledge level of the staff? How successful would new treatment strategies and implementation of new order sets be if basic knowledge regarding diabetes management was inconsistent or outdated? Therefore, I decided that a survey of nursing knowledge should be conducted prior to implementing a full-blown educational program. Knowledge obtained from the survey would guide the development of an evidence-based educational program for staff nurses.

I went back to the literature. Much to my delight and surprise, an existing tool that assesses diabetes knowledge of the medical-surgical nurse had been developed. I thought this would be easy: Contact the original author, obtain permission to use the tool, and conduct the research study. However, once I received the tool, I realized that components of the tool were based on standards of care almost 20 years old. Before I could ever conduct the study, I needed to revise the tool based on current American Diabetes Association standards, establish content validity with a panel of experts, perform pilot testing, further revise the tool based on initial results, and establish reliability over time. What had I gotten myself into?

FEELINGS AFTER CONDUCTING RESEARCH

The process is never-ending. Even when I thought the project was moving along, there were challenges placed in front of me. I am still conducting the research project, but it has taken a different avenue. The initial plan to assess basic diabetes knowledge of the staff nurse has led me to first revise the diabetes knowledge assessment tool and to determine the psychometrics of the revised tool. When this phase of the project is over, there will be other avenues for additional research, or possibilities for publishing and presenting the results.

The process of conducting research has given me a deeper appreciation for evidence-based practice and the research process. I have a deeper appreciation for the time and rigor needed to successfully develop and implement a research project. I also have developed a stronger professional sense of obligation to precept graduate nursing students in their research projects. I more fully understand and appreciate the IRB process, which always seeks to protect the rights of research participants. I have a deep, thankful appreciation for the individuals who mentored me when I started my research project and who have been supporting me throughout this endeavor. So, what have I learned?

ADVICE

1. Don't procrastinate! Get started! Start writing as you are implementing the project; this will help prevent you from omitting key information in the final project.
2. Start with something simple, something that you have strong clinical interest in and that will impact patient care. This will become your driving force when you have moments of discouragement.
3. Find an experienced researcher who can help guide you through the process the entire way, from development of the idea, to writing the proposal, to submitting the proposal to the IRB, to implementing the study. Schedule regular meetings with this researcher.

4. Find an experienced statistician up front when developing the project. He or she can suggest the appropriate sample size, the selection process, and statistical methods for data analysis.

5. Learn how to use the most advanced technological applications for performing literature searches, categorizing data, organizing data, and developing a bibliography. Investing the time up front will save you time in the long run.

6. Develop a written timeline to achieve specific project goals. Be prepared to adjust timelines when other pressing projects approach, but always go back to the project.

7. Engage the support of key physicians, nursing colleagues, graduate students, staff nurses, managers, and the chief nursing officer. These individuals will go to bat for you when the going gets tough.

8. Plan to dedicate specific time to the research project every week. Plan to invest lots and lots of additional time.

9. Revisit the literature from time to time to investigate whether more recent studies have been published and whether they are applicable to your research project.

10. Always check in with the experts to ensure that you are on the right track. Be prepared to take a less traveled, more difficult route as Robert Frost so eloquently stated in his poem, "The Road Not Taken."

So the journey continues, from being mentored to mentoring staff nurses and graduate students in the research process, from being a novice in research to an advanced beginner and sharing that knowledge with the next generation of nurses. Please read on to the next chapter for a few thoughts from my mentee, Jocelyn Holmes.

Acknowledgment: The author would like to acknowledge Dr. Janice Phillips, PhD, RN, FAAN, nurse researcher, University of Chicago Medical Center, for her expertise, guidance, and unending support for us as novice researchers.

I Can't Believe It's Research

Jocelyn D. Holmes

In the winter of 2006, I was in the midst of taking classes for my graduate degree, clinical nurse specialist in adult health. That semester, I was scheduled to take Research in Adult Health. I was exposed to nursing research while pursuing my undergraduate nursing degree. Nursing research was not my favorite subject—here we go again, ad hocs, and quantitative versus qualitative research. All kinds of things crossed my mind: *I've gotten all As thus far, I may have to settle for a B this time. I know I can at least get a B in this class. Tuesdays and Thursdays, here we go, I can't believe it's time for nursing research!*

During the course, we had a couple of guest speakers. One in particular was our nurse researcher, who is well known throughout our hospital (University of Chicago Medical Center). She spoke about how to develop a proposal. I kept thinking, *I cannot do this! I will not be writing a proposal, this is just too much work!* I remember thinking to myself, *How could one person be so excited about research? She is so smart! What do I have to do to get a PhD in nursing?* I continued to listen to her lecture; she also discussed the importance of African Americans impacting nursing research. *Sounds like a good idea. Can I do it? She is encouraging. OK, I'm going to follow the guidelines that she has given us. I am going to write this proposal. I am going to make my impact on nursing research.*

Days go by. It's time to hand in the research proposal to complete the assignment. I'm looking at the examples. I'm looking in the book. *You know what? Something's just not clicking here. The nurse researcher made it sound so easy. I'm going to put this paper together and say a prayer. It is what it is.*

I didn't get the desired result on that paper. *I am really going to try to do better next time*, I thought to myself. Needless to say, I said a lot of prayers. I earned an A in that course. God is good, all the time, all the time GOD IS GOOD!!!

In winter 2007, I entered my last semester of graduate school. The last course to complete was Adult Health Internship and Project. We were asked to find our own clinical preceptors. *What a task this is going to be!* I e-mailed my clinical nurse specialist (CNS) for general medicine for her assistance. I asked her if she had any colleagues who were willing to be a preceptor. To my surprise, she was looking for someone to precept to fulfill her obligations as a CNS. In addition, she was working on a research project to add to her growth as a CNS. *I can't believe it's time for research, again!*

The CNS asked if I would like to work with her as a research assistant. "Yes, I would like to be involved," I stated. *Now why did I say yes? I don't want any part of research. Nursing research doesn't like me, and I don't like it!* I said yes because this was an excellent opportunity that I could not pass up. *Hopefully, this will help me understand research better, and maybe I'll even like it.*

She shared her research with me (diabetes knowledge assessment among medical-surgical nurses). She shared articles, her review of the literature, and her abstract. I thought, *Oh my goodness, this is so overwhelming. You have to be so smart to put all this together!* I did my own review of literature, and I compared the articles with my CNS. *OK*, I thought, *I must be on the right track; I have a lot of the same articles that she has already found.* I actually went to the library to obtain some articles! I've always been lucky enough to retrieve my articles online. The next step with this research project was to complete online training on the protection of human subjects. *I am really going to go through with this.* And so I continued my research journey. I obtained verbal consents from staff nurses and administered the Diabetes Basic Knowledge Tool to staff. I learned a lot from this research project, including the importance of obtaining a mentor to assist with the flow of the project, the process of submitting a research proposal, and the impact of the research on nursing practice, my colleagues, and my institution. Working on this research project also allowed me to give input on new physician order sets for better diabetes patient management. In addition, I obtained the idea to do a needs assessment for diabetes as my final graduate project. I discovered that our adult inpatient units were in dire need of diabetes education in-services, updated education materials, and a diabetes educator. *Guess what? This is nursing research!*

Three months after graduate school, I was offered a role in developing a pilot project to improve the care of elder patients and confused patients in the inpatient setting. *I can't believe its research, AGAIN!* Of course, I immediately said yes to this opportunity. I would be crazy not to do it! With the assistance of our CNS and my care center director, an observation care program was developed based on the concepts of the Hospital Elder Life Program (HELP) and the Nurses Improving Care for Health System Elders (NICHE) program. We developed evidence-based delirium protocols for use with elderly patients with dementia and/or delirium. In addition to the program development, I was asked to begin writing about the observation care program and to prepare a research proposal. *What? Didn't they know that I vowed last year that I would never do a research proposal? Am I going to do it? Of course, I'm not crazy! I don't know what I'm doing, but I will utilize my resources, our CNS, our institution's nurse researcher, and my clinical director. We will get it done! Nursing research at its best! Maybe research is for me after all!*

Acknowledgment: The author would like to acknowledge Dr. Janice Phillips, PhD, RN, FAAN, nurse researcher, University of Chicago Medical Center, for her expertise, guidance, and unending support for us as novice researchers.

Diabetes Knowledge Assessment Among Medical-Surgical Nurses

Jocelyn D. Holmes, MS, RN

Purpose: The original aim of this study was to assess the basic knowledge level of the inpatient registered nurse regarding diabetes and diabetes management in the hospital. The results of the study would be used to develop ongoing nursing education programs in diabetes mellitus, including the basal-bolus insulin management concept. While initiating the study, the purpose changed to revising the existing knowledge assessment tool based on current standards of care for diabetes management and then testing the revised tool to determine content validity and reliability.

Design: This descriptive study was designed to assess nursing knowledge of diabetes and diabetes management in the acute care setting.

Methods: Permission to revise the Diabetes Basic Knowledge Tool (DBKT) was obtained from the original author. After reviewing the literature, specific questions that did not reflect contemporary evidence-based practice were deleted, and additional questions were developed to reflect current American Diabetes Association standards of care.

Results:

Content validity: Content validity was tested by a panel of experts composed of five certified diabetic educators. Eight questions that did not achieve minimum agreement among the content experts were deleted. The revised DBKT had a total of 41 questions, and the final content validity index was calculated at 0.92 (range 0.8–1.0).

Reliability: The DBKT was administered to 112 RNs to assess reliability estimates. The calculated Cronbach's alpha coefficient of the DBKT was 0.71.

Readability testing: The Flesch-Kincaid Grade Level score in Microsoft Word was calculated at a grade level of 9.5. The Flesch Reading Ease was calculated at 52.1%. Thirteen percent of the sentences were written in the passive voice. Thus, the revised DBKT was written at a reading level appropriate to the registered nurse who had completed a minimum of 2 years of college education.

Conclusions: Additional psychometric testing of the tool is needed to establish further reliability. A test-retest is in progress, and, when completed, the Cronbach's alpha coefficients will be calculated to ascertain test-retest reliability. The final revised DBKT will be administered to medical-surgical nurses to identify nursing knowledge of inpatient diabetes management.

(2007)

CHAPTER 21

The Never-Ending Research Study

Sharon Kimball

A few years before we began our unit-based research project, I attended a nursing research conference and was frustrated by the lack of any research "applicable" to my practice. There were many interesting speakers and poster presentations, but there was no connection to my day-to-day work. I also saw no link between the doctorally prepared researchers and me. They were for researching, I was for implementing, but the two areas were not anywhere near a connection!

To encourage research and prepare for Magnet application, our hospital brought in a consultant. She presented a model to us that turned nursing research upside down. Guided by a research mentor, usually a nurse with an advanced degree, the staff nurses decided on their research question, conducted a lit review, designed the study, and carried it out. The consultant provided support throughout the process and in the analysis of the data. The end product was a completed research study that would impact the practice of the nurses working on the unit.

To decide on a research question, the unit-based research model leads the staff nurses through a brainstorming and then a winnowing process. We had many, many ideas. But after evaluating each idea using criteria set by the model, we landed on a question about discharge medication teaching.

As an acute rehabilitation unit, everything we do for patients is geared toward preparing them for discharge. However, we felt that we sort of "threw" their discharge medication teaching at them as they were heading out the door, and we wanted to improve this process. Rehabilitation patients are accustomed to a set daily therapy schedule. We wondered, if we scheduled a medication teaching time, like a set physical therapy time, would the patients learn more? Would they take the teaching more seriously? Would they treat their session with us with as much respect as they treat the session with their physical or occupational therapist?

We were also unhappy with the format of our printed medication information sheets. We felt that the print was too small and that the sheets were too crowded with information, making it difficult for the patients to easily comprehend what was vital for them to know about their medication versus what was not.

Because of the small size of our unit, 18 beds, it took us a year to design our study and then 8 months to collect the data. We had consistent participation in the unit's research group; every nurse who started at the beginning of this project was still participating at the end! As we moved through the process, we became more than a little burnt out with data collection and trying to identify subjects. It was frustrating when possible subjects were not signed up because we got busy on the unit, thus lengthening our data collection. Or you signed up a subject, did the pretest, did the teaching, and then—oops! You were off the next day, and the person designated to do the posttest did not get the message to do it. Another subject bites the dust!

For some of our researchers, it was hard to stick to the strict design of our study, particularly as we got closer to the end. They would think, "that patient would be perfect for Group 3" instead of sticking with the random assignment. We had to have a talk or two about that! Sometimes, after 7 months of data collection, you would think, "Well, he *almost* meets the inclusion criteria. . ." We stayed true to our study in the end, no matter how tempting it might have been to speed up the process!

Overall, though, it was a positive experience. Now that we have finished slogging through the data collection and almost have a completed manuscript that we are going to try to submit for publication, some nurses are asking, "What are we going to do for our next study?"

Through this guided process, we learned a lot about reading research articles with a critical eye, how research studies are set up, how data are collected, and how to successfully complete a study. We learned how to use the hospital library's online tools to do a lit search. We learned what the heck the "IRB" is. We didn't know any of this at the start, but we supported each other, stayed engaged, and took it one step at a time. We also owe a lot to a very supportive unit manager and research mentor. We found that people are very eager to share their knowledge and provide guidance, if you only ask them. We now routinely ask, "What's the evidence?" around our practice.

By the way, because of the influence of our nursing research consultant and the others involved in supporting us through this research project, I went back to school and completed my master's as a clinical nurse leader. I moved off the rehab unit and into a new position. We are still working on our study, and the manuscript is almost complete!

Acknowledgment: This study would never have been attempted without the teamwork, humor, and commitment of a great group of rehabilitation nurses: Gail Buck, Debora Goldstein, Kris Kalman-Yearout, Elena Largaespada, Lauren Logan, and Diane Stebbins. I would like to acknowledge the expertise and guidance of Lisa Halvorsen, PhD, RN, and Marianne Chulay, DNSc, RN. Without Marianne's practical step-by-step research model, we never would have made this journey.

Testing a Teaching Appointment and Geragogy-Based Approach to Increase Patient Medication Knowledge at Discharge

Sharon Kimball, MS, RN, CNL, CRRN

This study was conducted on an 18-bed acute rehabilitation unit that is part of a 483-bed not-for-profit hospital in the Pacific Northwest. The study was approved by the institutional review board for the health system.

Purpose: To evaluate the effectiveness of the geragogy approach to teaching about discharge medications and a scheduled appointment for discharge teaching on patient or family member knowledge of, and confidence with, administration of discharge medications.

Study Design: A pretest-posttest experimental design was used to compare three different methods of patient or family member medication teaching at patient discharge from an acute rehabilitation unit. Subjects were randomly assigned to one of three different teaching methods: patient or family member appointment with use of a geragogy format approach for presentation of medication information (experimental); use of a geragogy format approach for presentation of medication information (experimental); or usual nurse patient/family member teaching (control). The dependent variables were the difference in pretest and posttest scores on a medication knowledge test and ratings of confidence in administering discharge medications, as well as a posttest rating of satisfaction with medication information received by the patient or family member. Random assignment to groups was done using a computer-generated randomization sequence.

Methods: Using a convenience sample of patients or family members, a randomized experimental study design was used to compare three different methods for teaching about discharge medications: geragogy format with a scheduled time for teaching, geragogy format alone, and standard format alone. Prior to discharge, subjects were taught with the assigned teaching method and evaluated on the following variables: pretest and posttest knowledge of the discharge medication, pretest and posttest confidence with discharge medication administration, and satisfaction with teaching method. Data were analyzed with analysis of variance with two factors—teaching method and subject type—and Scheffe's multiple comparison test, with $p < 0.05$ considered significant.

Results: A total of 66 subjects ($N = 41$ patients; $N = 25$ family members) were studied. No significant differences were found between the three teaching methods, but a significant difference was found between patients' and family members' confidence level with administering discharge medications ($p = 0.002$). Family members had significantly lower confidence levels before the teaching sessions than did patients, and confidence levels after the education were similar for both groups.

Conclusion: This study found that family members had significantly lower confidence levels in administering discharge medications before education than did patients. The use of the geragogy format for teaching about discharge medications and the use of a scheduled time to provide the educational session did not significantly improve medication knowledge. Satisfaction with the teaching method was similar for all three teaching methods. These findings indicate that the caregiver's confidence level in administering discharge medications improves with discharge medication teaching more so than the patient's, perhaps because nurses provide incremental teaching about medications to patients over time. Because of the type of patients admitted to an acute rehabilitation unit, the patient may also have an inflated sense of ability based on pride or the physiology of his or her diagnosis. Caregiver role transition could also be a factor.

(2007)

Getting Step-Down Staff "Stuck On" Research

Katherine Nagy

Many of the nurses on our pulmonary step-down unit are "mature and experienced"—in other words, part of the over-40 crowd and steadfast believers in the way "nursing used to be." I am the clinical nurse specialist responsible for mentoring this seasoned staff (with whom I worked side by side for 20 years) on entrance into the world of research and evidence-based practice. To say the least, this venture has been challenging and has required me to be flexible and to persevere.

Having recently finished graduate school, I was eager to spread the word on creating more of a nursing science through research. I realized that the only way to get my staff on board would be through gaining their interest, recognizing their strengths, and assuring them that their efforts would improve patient care.

Multidisciplinary rounding (MDR) is routinely performed in our intensive care unit (ICU). All members of the healthcare team participate in the daily rounding. Many of the ICU patients are eventually transferred to our pulmonary step-down unit. Traditionally, there has been little formalized team care planning after the transfer. Because of the documented success of interdisciplinary care and the emphasis on research in our hospital, I approached the nurse manager with an idea for a study. After gaining her support, I posed a question to the staff leadership group: Could we improve any patient outcomes if we continued MDR on our unit? This thought sparked an interest among the group. After a thorough literature review, institutional review board acceptance, and collaboration with our nurse researcher, I took the lead in designing a pilot study that would describe the MDR on complex patients in a pulmonary step-down unit.

The experienced nurses were responsible for leading the biweekly rounding and documenting on a checklist (designed in collaboration by all of us). The less experienced nurses caring for the patients enhanced their critical thinking and problem-solving skills through the interaction with the expert staff. Respiratory therapy was the only discipline other than nursing that agreed to participate. Although disappointing, this didn't stop us, and the study was completed after 2 months.

How did we keep the momentum going? Through positive reinforcement and open communication. There were many times when a nurse would say, "I don't have time," or "What good is this doing?" After pointing out some examples of potential benefits, including reduced ventilator days, improved quality outcomes, and more timely discharges, staff interest was easily redirected.

We presented our preliminary findings at our hospital's Nursing Day of Inquiry. Other nurses from the hospital had many questions, and this interest provoked renewed excitement for our research. We plan to continue this study and actually examine outcomes (as opposed to our pilot, which described the rounding process). Who knows, maybe rounding will be incorporated into other patient care areas based on our findings. This alone is enough incentive for the nurses on the step-down unit to remain "stuck on research"!

What is my advice to other nurses? Find a topic that you are interested in, seek the guidance and support of experts, and jump in. There is no more rewarding feeling than knowing that you made a difference, not only for your own patients, but by adding your findings to nursing science and potentially impacting patients everywhere!

Acknowledgment: The author would like to acknowledge Glenda Kelman, PhD, APRN, BC, for her encouragement and support of my research projects. It was a privilege to have studied under her in graduate school, and I am fortunate that she remains my greatest professional nursing mentor!

Multidisciplinary Rounding on Complex Pulmonary Step-Down Patients in a Community Hospital

Katherine Nagy, MS, APRN, BC; Linda Michalak, MS, RN;
Alice Abrams, BS, RN; and June Teets, RN

Purpose/Problem: The purpose of this study was to describe multidisciplinary rounding (MDR) on complex patients in a pulmonary step-down unit. Multidisciplinary care is a method of providing quality, seamless care to patients in the hospital setting. Positive patient outcomes are achieved through communication, collaboration, and shared expertise between members of the healthcare team. Studies have supported the use of collaborative rounding to improve patient outcomes in critical care areas (Halm, et al., 2003). Daily patient rounding is already a standard practice in the hospital's intensive care unit. Patients transferred from critical care areas to 4 G remain complex and in need of a multidisciplinary plan of care.

Design/Methods: After obtaining institutional review board consent, participants ($N = 20$) were chosen by the healthcare team based on criteria including, but not exclusive of, diagnosis, respiratory needs, acuity level, and discharge plans. Twice weekly, members of the healthcare team reviewed the patient's record/plan of care and collaborated on determining individualized patient outcomes and goals. The rounding process enabled a comprehensive plan of care to be established and assisted in determining daily priorities. Information was documented on a checklist developed by the nursing staff. The study ran from August 3 to September 28, 2007, with 52 rounding sessions completed on 20 complex patients.

Results: Twenty-one percent of the unit's patients were complex. Biweekly MDRs were completed 82% of the time, with 14% of these rounds documented in the medical record (100% were documented on the rounding checklist). One of two identified staff nurse experts (RN 3, RN 4) led each MDR. The composition of the potential team members was RN 3 (58%), RN 4 (85%), operations manager (35%), clinical nurse specialist (25%), staff nurse (79%), and respiratory therapist

(100%). The most commonly identified patient goals were discharge needs (52%), weaning (19%), increased activity (19%), and end of life care (10%).

Conclusion: The findings were disseminated to 4 G nursing staff and the respiratory therapy department. The rounding checklist will be modified based on findings. Medical record documentation will be reviewed with staff. This study will be extended to examine the potential relationship between multidisciplinary rounding, length of weaning, activity levels, discharge disposition, and length of stay.

REFERENCES

Halm, M., Gagner, S., Goering, M., Sabo, J., Smith, M., & Zaccagnini, M. (2003). Interdisciplinary rounds: Impact on patients, families, and staff. *Clinical Nurse Specialist, 17*(3), 133–142.

CHAPTER 23

The Spark That Triggered My Research Reaction

Denise Cedeno

Like many of my colleagues, my major exposure to research occurred through college courses and special assignments. At that time, my motivation to do research was to complete assignments. Today, I think quite differently. I am involved in research now for the same reason that I became a nurse: to help people! My most recent opportunity came while working as a charge nurse at a community hospital in upstate New York.

I was approached by our infection control nurse. She wanted to know why the nosocomial urinary tract infection rate for our unit was one of the highest in the hospital. I didn't have an answer. That bothered me. I thought about it for a while and then asked myself, "Is the high nosocomial urinary tract infection rate on our unit accurate, or is it a reflection of deviation in the procedure for collecting urine specimens?" To find an answer, I conducted a study of the procedures used on our unit to collect specimens for routine urinalysis and urine cultures for patients who could void and for patients who had indwelling urinary catheters. At the time, I wasn't thinking about research; I was only trying to find an answer to an important question that affected quality patient care. I found the answer to my question and shared my findings with the unit staff, and practice was changed based on my study.

One day while participating in annual nursing reorientation, one of the presenters was talking about evidence-based practice and nursing research. It suddenly occurred to me that I had done a research project! Not only that, my findings were used to change practice! Wow! One does not have to be a rocket scientist to conduct research, one can be a nurse—who takes care of patients.

Based on my experience, I feel that nursing research should not be feared, because a nurse can start with a simple study and advance as time goes on. Research findings can create more questions and more research opportunities. Resources and support are available through the hospital, libraries, the computer, and many other sources. All it took was a spark to trigger my research reaction, so don't be afraid to give it a try. It's worth it!

Acknowledgment: I would like to acknowledge Fran Anderson, PhD, RN, for her patience, support, and encouragement to me in my pursuit of doing research at Lourdes Hospital.

Decreasing Nosocomial Urinary Tract Infections

Denise Cedeno, BS, RN

Purpose: Hospital-acquired urinary tract infections (UTIs) contribute substantially to patient morbidity, mortality, and healthcare costs and are the most frequently occurring nosocomial (hospital-acquired) infections in hospitals in the United States and abroad. At our hospital, one such infection increases length of stay for a patient by 3.6 days and costs approximately $5,516 per episode. This was unacceptable in terms of quality patient care. The purpose of this study was to answer the question, Is the high nosocomial urinary tract infection rate on our unit accurate, or is it a reflection of deviation in the procedure for collecting urine specimens?

Design: A purposive sample of 22 registered nurses and patient care assistants were interviewed.

Methods: Each staff member was asked the following questions: (1) How do you collect a urine specimen for a urine culture or urinalysis on male and female patients who are able to void? (2) How do you collect urine specimens for a urine culture or urinalysis on male and female patients with a Foley catheter? When a staff member described the correct procedure, he or she was congratulated. When a staff member described an incorrect procedure, he or she was reminded of the correct method based on evidence in the literature and the hospital's evidence-based policy and procedure for collecting urine specimens. Data were analyzed using descriptive statistics.

Results: The data showed that staff used the correct procedure to collect a voided specimen for urine culture only 8% of the time. In addition, they used the correct procedure to collect a voided specimen for routine urinalysis only 25% of the time. In contrast, when a patient had a Foley catheter in place, staff used the correct procedure to collect a specimen for urine culture 70% of the time, and for a routine urinalysis, 82% of the time.

Conclusions: The findings from this study were the basis for development of a urinary care bundle at our hospital. Nursing staff and physician education includes handwashing and implementation of the urinary care bundle, which incorporates the following: (1) toileting dependent and incontinent patients every 2 hours, and routine perineal and incontinent care; (2) justification for insertion of Foleys (specific reason, not convenience) and daily assessment of continued need; (3) proper Foley insertion procedure (handwashing, sterile technique, securing catheter, correct size and type, silver lined); (4) proper specimen-collection technique; and (5) care and maintenance of Foleys (i.e., bag handling with ambulation, bed, chair, transport). Since implementation of the urinary care bundle on our unit, the nosocomial UTI rate on the unit has decreased steadily from a high of 11.14.

(2006)

CHAPTER 24

Did I Just Agree to Do Research?

Kathleen Fitzgerald

My first exposure to nursing research was in graduate school in 1992. Along with a fellow student, I had done a research study on patients requiring 1:1 sitter observation at New England Medical Center in Boston. Research was a requirement of the graduate program. I never thought I would be doing research again during my career as a nurse.

One day at Winchester Hospital, I was walking down the hallway to my office. I passed by a conference room where our Magnet coordinator was meeting with our Magnet consultant. They called me in and asked, "Do you think you could replicate this study on discharge planning?" My initial response was "Sure I can," but when I said that, I did not realize the magnitude of what I had just committed to. Once I returned to my office and looked at the published study further, it dawned on me: *Oh my god, I just committed to doing a nursing research study.* The panic set in. I was convinced that I would fail miserably.

Winchester Hospital was just starting on its Magnet journey in the spring of 2002. One of the requirements was nursing research, which we did not have in place at the time. I knew how important achieving this recognition was to the institution as a whole, and I needed to be a team player and do my part. I am the director of case management, so it was a logical request that I replicate a study on discharge planning.

I was initially afraid that I had forgotten everything I had learned in graduate school about doing research, but I was fortunate to have a great mentor who took charge of the nursing research process. I was not alone; I had support through the entire research process.

The hospital was extremely vested in the Magnet journey. Everyone was determined to succeed, so senior leadership ensured that we had the support and resources we needed to achieve Magnet status.

Shortly after being asked to do nursing research, a series of meetings was put together to give us direction with the research process. This was extremely helpful because it provided us with the resources and up-to-date information regarding the research process. The hospital contracted with a statistician and two university faculty nursing researchers who were at our disposal throughout the entire process. The hospital also has an excellent medical staff library with a full-time librarian who was available to do our literature searches and obtain copies of the articles we would need.

My mentor through the research process made sure I stayed on a timeline. We met regularly, and she was there for every step of the process to make sure I was on the right track and had all my questions answered.

Once I was reeducated on the research process, I did the literature search. I completed my research proposal and went to the institutional review board (IRB) in December 2002 for approval. Initially I was rather intimidated by all the people in the room whom I needed to present to, but I was put at great ease once I listened to a few proposals that were presented before mine. The members of the IRB were very welcoming and actually made the process fairly painless.

Once I had my IRB approval, I contacted the authors of the research study that I was about to replicate to ask their permission to use their data collection tools. They responded immediately and granted me permission to use their tools and offered to be available to me for any further questions I might have while going through the research process.

My next step was the survey that was distributed to the nursing staff. I needed to first educate the nurse managers and the nursing staff about the discharge planning survey and its purpose. I was able to elicit the support of the staff development clinical nurse specialists to help educate the staff nurses about the survey. The staff nurses were very receptive to the survey because they understood that it was part of the nursing research process needed for our Magnet quest.

I spent several months doing data collection via chart review and reviewing our inpatient Press Ganey surveys on patient satisfaction. Once the data were collected and the surveys returned, I was given access to secretarial support that tabulated responses and put the data into Excel spreadsheets. These spreadsheets were then e-mailed to our statistician. I met with the statistician to review the data and the purpose of the study. He came back with an analysis of the data and met with me again to go over the data analysis.

Now it was time to form the conclusions, write the research article, and publish.

I set my goals high and sent letters to many top nursing journals, all of which expressed interest. I sent my research manuscript to each journal one by one, but I was not prepared for how difficult this process would be. I have had three rejections and one that wanted me to incorporate a nursing theorist into the research. I discussed this with my mentor, and we chose not to do it at that time. I was in the process of choosing the next journal to submit to when I learned of this book—*Real Stories of Nursing Research: The Quest for Magnet Recognition*—being published. I decided to submit my story here.

Since I began my research journey, Winchester Hospital has been successful in developing a research council that was nursing only at the beginning but has since become multidisciplinary. This council supports all staff who are doing research at the hospital.

I have had the opportunity to present my research to the Nursing Leadership Council at Winchester Hospital, and my research was accepted for a poster presentation at a national nursing conference this June in Washington DC, which was shocking news. I did not expect it to be accepted.

In the beginning, I did not think I had the time or the support to do a research project, but I was wrong. I found that if you booked a set time into your calendar, the work did get done. In the beginning, you do feel overwhelmed and think, *Will I be able to do this or ever see an end product?* I was extremely fortunate to have all the support that I had with the research process, which essentially was the key to my success. It was important that the topic I was researching had meaning and importance to me because that kept me focused and vested in accomplishing a finished manuscript.

My advice to other nurses: Nursing research can be scary if you have never done it before, but if you are working in an environment with great supports and structure, it is achievable and not as bad as you think it may be. Seek out those who know the research process, and find a mentor to help you stay focused and on track. Know who your resources are before you start. It takes a long time, but in the end, the results are quite personally and professionally rewarding. I would recommend choosing a subject that you are passionate about; you will enjoy and easily comprehend the literature review process and find it easy to formulate your conclusions. Once the manuscript is complete, attempt to publish. Do not give up; it takes time. Also, present what you have done to your fellow nursing colleagues and get the recognition you deserve.

Acknowledgments: I would like to acknowledge Dr. Kathleen Beyerman from Winchester Hospital, Winchester, Massachusetts, for her guidance through the research process, and Nasreen Sulaimon from Aga Khan University Hospital, Karachi, Pakistan, for providing the instrument she used in her discharge planning study.

Discharge Planning Perspectives of Patients and Nurses

Kathleen Fitzgerald, MSN, RN, ACM

Purpose: The objective of this study is to evaluate patient satisfaction, nurse perceptions and knowledge, and nursing documentation of the discharge planning process. Discharge planning is a vital part of the continuum of patient care. It begins on admission and is a collaborative process between the healthcare team, patient, and family. Parkes and Shepperd (2000) defined *discharge planning* as "the development of an individualized discharge plan for the patient before leaving the hospital, with the aim of containing costs and improving patient outcomes." Nurses play an essential role in the discharge planning process because of their direct involvement in patient care and their ongoing assessment of patients' needs throughout their hospitalizations. A study by Lalani and Gulzar (2001) found that nurses had a limited understanding of the concept of discharge planning. The study strongly suggested that the nurses' role and their knowledge of discharge planning needed to be strengthened and reinforced. Nurses must realize the importance of discharge planning to provide cost-effective, high-quality nursing care.

Patient satisfaction is a vital outcome measurement in health care; patients expect high-quality health care. Healthcare providers are presently challenged by increasing costs and shorter lengths of stay for patients in the acute care setting. This challenge reinforces the need for making discharge planning an integral part of each patient's hospitalization. A pilot study found that it is feasible to use patient evaluation as a measure of outcomes in discharge planning. Their study concluded that health outcomes, as defined by consumers, could provide a measure for evaluating service delivery and need to be further used by nurses involved in planning care. Parkes and Shepperd (2000) found evidence that patients who received discharge planning had increased patient satisfaction. Therefore, nurses must understand the importance of their role in discharge planning.

The purpose of this descriptive study was to:

- explore staff nurses' knowledge and perceptions of discharge planning;
- examine nurses' practices regarding discharge planning;

- identify ways to strengthen nursing's role in discharge planning; and
- evaluate patients' satisfaction with the discharge planning process.

Methods: The exploratory, descriptive study at Winchester Hospital (WH), a 200-bed community hospital north of Boston, was based on research conducted at the Aga Khan University Hospital in Pakistan.

The study was designed to provide perspectives from nurses and patients about the discharge planning process. The comprehensiveness of discharge planning was evaluated by conducting an audit of the patient's medical record. Nurses' knowledge and perceptions of discharge planning were obtained by having staff nurses complete a discharge-planning questionnaire. Patients' perceptions of discharge planning were obtained through a patient satisfaction survey.

Subjects: This IRB-approved study drew nurse participants from the intensive care unit (ICU) and medical-surgical units at WH. It included full- and part-time registered nurses who work days or evenings, but not night nurses or per diems.

Patient participants included all ICU and medical-surgical patients who were discharged during a specified time period and who completed an inpatient Press Ganey survey.

WH obtained informed consent from the nurses who participated in the written survey questionnaire.

Instruments: Instruments included a demographic data collection sheet, the Discharge Planning Questionnaire for Nurses (DPQN), the Chart Audit Tool, and the Inpatient Press Ganey Patient Satisfaction Survey.

Discharge Planning Questionnaire for Nurses: The DPQN was developed by Lalani and Gulzar (2001) for their study, "Nurses' Role in Patients' Discharge Planning at the Aga Khan University Hospital, Pakistan." Three nurses took part after content validity was determined by a senior research faculty member. Modifications were made, and the instrument was used with the 15 research participants in their study. The parts of the instrument used in this study were statements answered using a 5-point Likert scale. Open-ended questions were eliminated.

WH duplicated, with permission, the nursing questionnaire used by Lalani and Gulzar and then added seven more questions (Questions 13 and 14 were developed by WH to see how nursing perceived the role of case management, and Questions 15–19 were the same Press Ganey questions that patients were asked regarding patient satisfaction with discharge). For reporting purposes, the categories in the Likert-type scale were combined into two units: *agree* and *disagree. Don't know* was kept as a separate category.

Questions covered such topics as:

- Efficacy
- Importance

- Physician involvement
- Family involvement
- Timing of discharge planning
- Orientation to discharge planning
- Role of case managers
- Role of staff nurses

Inpatient Press Ganey Patient Satisfaction Survey: The Inpatient Press Ganey Patient Satisfaction Survey (IPGPSS) is a patient satisfaction survey used in 797 hospitals in the United States. Questions on discharge planning include:

- Extent to which you felt ready to be discharged
- Speed of discharge process after you were told you could go home
- Instructions given about how to care for yourself at home
- Help with arranging home care services (if needed)
- How well coordinated your discharge was from the hospital

The IPGPSS was first used in 1987 and was revised in 1997. Face, content, and consensus validities were established by the client advisory committee. In 2002, the survey was subjected to another study and revalidated. In this 5-point Likert scale, the questions had little or no variation, nor were they found to be too highly correlated with other questions (Press Ganey, 2002).

Both convergent validity and discriminant validity were demonstrated. The questionnaire shows high levels of predictive validity. All nine scales exceeded the stringent .70 standard for reliable measures. The Cronbach's alpha for the entire questionnaire is .98, confirming the instrument's high internal consistency and reliability. The Flesch-Kincaid Index confirms the questions at a fifth- to sixth-grade reading level.

Chart Audit Tool: The Chart Audit Tool was used to assess the documentation of discharge planning in the patient record. It includes assessing the following documents for evidence of discharge planning:

- Nursing notes
- Nursing assessment forms
- Nursing care plan
- Nursing discharge instruction sheet

Results:

Demographics

Descriptive statistics were used to describe the two populations—nurses and patients (**Table 24-1** and **Table 24-2**). Correlation coefficients were done to evaluate the relationship between some demographic data and survey response items. The study hospital surveyed registered nurses. The mean age

Table 24-1   Demographic Variables of Nurses

	(*n*)	%
Registered nurse (RN)	(42)	100%
Registered midwives	(0)	0%
Female nurses	(41)	97.6%
Male nurses	(1)	2.4%
Age (mean)	39.5	
Years of experience (mean)	14.7	

Table 24-2   Demographic Variables of Patients

	N = 314
Male	41%
Female	59%
Age (average)	66.4 years
Previous admission	64%
Length of stay	3.6 days
Insured	98.7%

of the nursing staff is 39.5 years old, and the staff is 97.6% female. The nurses' work experience averages 14.7 years.

The patient population was split—41% male and 59% female—with a mean age of 66.4 years. A majority of the patients (64%) had been hospitalized before at WH. The average length of stay of the sample was 3.6 days, and 98.7% were insured.

Nurses' Knowledge and Perceptions Regarding Discharge Planning
      All nurse participants agreed that discharge planning is an important role
of nurses. A total of 92.6% of the nurses agreed that they, as staff nurses, participated effectively in the discharge planning process. There was a similar
response of 68.3% as to whether physicians were actively involved in discharge
planning. A high perception (90.2%) was reported of families being involved in
their relative's discharge plan. Only 83% of the nurses felt that discharge planning began early on their units. Nurses noted that they did not have adequate
time to plan for the discharge of their patients. Over 95% of the nurses believed
that documentation of all discharge activities must be done on all patients. The
nurses (90.5%) felt strongly that discharge planning was an essential part of the
nursing care plan Only 45.5% of the nurses felt that they had adequate orientation to discharge planning.
      The questions added to the DPQN (Questions 13–19) were derived from the
IPGPSS. The nurses saw the discharge process as a collaborative effort, not the
sole responsibility of the case manager. The nurses were also asked the same
five questions that the patients were asked in relation to patient discharge. A

Table 24-3   Nurses' Knowledge and Perceptions Regarding Discharge Planning

Statements	Agree %
1. Discharge planning is an important role of nurses.	100%
2. On your unit, staff nurses participate effectively in discharge planning.	92.6%
3. Nurses on your unit regularly carry out the needs assessment for discharge planning.	82.5%
4. On your unit, most physicians are actively involved in discharge planning.	68.3%
5. On your unit, families are involved in their relative's discharge plan.	90.2%
6. Discharge planning begins early in the hospitalization.	83%
7. As a nurse, I don't have enough time to plan discharge for my patients.	54.7%

(Continued)

Table 24-3   *(Continued)*

Statements	Agree %
8. Overall, discharge planning in this hospital is carried out to meet patients' needs.	90.2%
9. Documentation of all discharge activities must be done on every patient.	95.2%
10. Discharge planning is an essential part of the patient's nursing care plan.	90.5%
11. Discharge planning is part of the nursing process.	100%
12. An appropriate orientation to discharge planning is provided for new staff members.	45.5%
13. Case managers are solely responsible for the discharge plan of all patients.	9.7%
14. Case managers work collaboratively with all members of the healthcare team to ensure positive patient outcomes on discharge.	97.6%
15. Patients I discharged felt ready to be discharged.	88.1%
16. Patients I discharged felt satisfied with the speed of the discharge process after they were told they could go home.	65.8%
17. Patients I discharged were satisfied with instructions given about how to care for themselves at home.	95%
18. Patients I discharged felt satisfied with the help in arranging home care services (if needed).	100%
19. Patients I discharged were satisfied with how well coordinated their discharge was from the hospital.	97.3%

majority (88.1%) of the nurses said that their patients felt ready for discharge but that the actual speed of the process could be improved. Overall, the nurses perceived that patients discharged were generally very satisfied with their home care discharge instructions, the arrangement of home care services, and the overall coordination of their discharge.

Patients' Perceptions of Discharge Planning

The study hospital collected the same descriptive statistics (e.g., percentages, frequencies, and variance) as Lalani and Gulzar (2001) to analyze the demographic variables of the patients' questionnaire. They also looked at the patients' perceptions of their satisfaction with the discharge process, whereas Lalani and Gulzar (2001) examined the patients' perceptions of their involvement in the discharge process. Overall, the patients who participated in the survey were satisfied with the discharge process. When asked whether the discharge instructions they received were helpful at home, 92% of the patients surveyed said that they were satisfied.

Documentation of Discharge Planning: The Chart Audit Tool was used to assess the documentation of discharge planning in the patient record at WH. The charts reviewed were of those patients who participated in the IPGPSS (n = 314 charts).

The four areas of documentation that were addressed were as follows:

1. Were the discharge planning needs documented on the initial nursing assessment?
2. Was there nursing documentation of discharge planning in the patient's progress notes?
3. Was there a completed nursing discharge instruction sheet in the medical record?
4. Was there documentation regarding discharge planning on the nursing care plan?

Table 24-4   Nurses' and Patients' Perceptions Regarding Their Satisfaction with Discharge Planning

	Nurses	Patients
Extent to which the patient felt ready to be discharged	88%	90%
Speed of the discharge process once you were told you could go home	65.8%	85%
Instructions given about how to care for yourself at home	90%	95%
Help with arranging home care services (if needed)	100%	90%
How well coordinated was your discharge from the hospital?	97.3%	90%

Of the four audit measures, two showed very high rates of documentation, and two measures showed much lower rates. Ninety-five percent of the time, there was nursing documentation of discharge planning in the patient progress notes (Audit Item 2) and a completed nursing discharge instruction sheet in the medical record (Audit Item 3). More than 58% of the time, there was an indication of discharge planning needs documented on the initial nursing assessment (Audit Item 1), and just over a third of the time (35.4%), there was documentation regarding discharge planning on the nursing care plan (Audit Item 4).

Conclusions: The findings from this study confirmed that the nurses had a good understanding of discharge planning and believed that it is an important part of the nursing process. They see themselves as active participants. Even though most nurses noted that it is important to start discharge planning on admission, only about 60% indicated discharge planning needs on the initial nursing admission assessment. The nurses were very compliant with the documentation of discharge instructions and in writing a discharge progress note, but they were not very compliant with documenting discharge planning on the nursing care plan. The nurses reported that they did not have enough time to plan for the discharge of their patients.

There are ways to strengthen the nurses' role in discharge planning. One is understanding what the patients say needs to be improved. Only 85% of the patients were satisfied with the speed of the discharge process once they were told that they could go home. Although this may seem adequate, it is below the threshold of acceptable scores at the study hospital. The nurses intuitively understood this. On the same item, they scored the speed of discharge at 65.8%—well below what the patients reported.

Table 24-5   Discharge Planning Documentation

Documentation form	$n = 314$ charts
Nursing assessment	58.6%
Progress notes	95%
Discharge instruction sheet	95%
Care plan	35.4%

There was also a 5- to 10-point difference in the views of nurses and patients about the adequacy of discharge instructions, help with arranging home care services, and the coordination of discharge. WH nurses rated their performance in these areas higher than the patients rated them. It is helpful for nurses to understand that they and their patients may have different views of discharge planning.

The charting showed low compliance with documenting discharge planning in the nursing assessment and nursing care plan. These data were collected before computers were used for record keeping. In general, there is reason to believe that nurses begin discharge planning early in the hospitalization, that they take an active role in it themselves, and that they involve families in the plan. The nurses believe that discharge planning is part of the nursing process and that new staff members do not receive adequate orientation. The nurses say it is important but that they do not get enough education on the topic. That discrepancy may be used as an opportunity for improvement in this vital component of the continuity of care.

REFERENCES

Lalani, N. S., & Gulzar, A. Z. (2001). Nurses' role in patients' discharge planning at the Aga Khan University Hospital, Pakistan. *Journal for Nurses in Staff Development, 17*(6), 314–319.

Parkes, J., & Shepperd, S. (2000). Discharge planning from hospital to home. *Cochrane Database System Revision*, (4). CD000313.

Press Ganey. (2002). *Press Ganey satisfaction measurement inpatient psychometrics.*

CHAPTER 25

How the Passion for Research Was Ignited: The Experience of One Novice Researcher

Mary Beth Strauss

Research, the very word, used to make me cringe and run the other way. It would instill panic in me and is the one reason that I chose my particular graduate program—it had no research requirement, and we only had to do a scholarly paper. How great was that? That was until I had done it, after this thing called Magnet came along

Now, we've all heard of Magnet Recognition, and as a part of nursing staff development, I was involved with gathering evidence for some of the initial standards (referred to as Forces). My department was responsible for working on a research standard. At the time of our initial application in the spring of 2002, I was working as a part-time nursing staff development specialist and as a staff nurse in our 200-bed not-for-profit community hospital. I was not a researcher. One afternoon, our director pulled a group of us together to look at the research standard and to brainstorm about how we could meet the requirements. The question posed to us was about possible research topics in the Department of Nursing. Everyone kind of looked around, and we talked about a few things. Then I came up with an idea of looking at our restraint use and determining if our restraint reduction initiative was effective in reducing restraint use. The meeting continued.

Shortly after our meeting, early in the evening before going home, the director walked into my office, sat down, and said to me, "Your research question is really the most plausible and logical one to go after." In the back of my mind, I was thinking, *Where is she going with this?* And then she hit me with, "What do you think about doing a research study on this topic?" I think I laughed nervously first and told her I didn't know how to do research and wouldn't even know where to begin. She very calmly told me, "We'll go step by step and use all our resources to ensure it gets done right. Why don't we just start with an overview of the literature and develop a good research question?" I accepted the challenge, she left the office, and I thought, *Oh no, what am I going to do?* It was late and nobody was around, so the following day, I immediately coerced my office mate and colleague into being my coinvestigator. I was not going to do this alone.

At our first meeting with our fearless leader, she had us develop a timeline. She assured us that it was very fluid, and she was right. We continually revised the timeline based on obstacles we encountered or because of other work commitments/priorities. A timeline was a wonderful tool and kept us to task. It was at this meeting that we were told that we had to fully intend to publish the research, "because isn't that why we do research?" In the back of my mind, I was thinking, *You've got to be kidding!*

And so our research journey began. In the back of my mind, I always kept thinking that this would never really happen; other things would take priority, this would be put aside for something better or just be forgotten. Well, soon it started to progress. We were at the IRB, then all of a sudden we were talking to a statistician, and then we were collecting data; this was going to happen. And happen it did. My coinvestigator and I completed the research study and submitted it for publication. In the end, we were not published, but there were wonderful learning points along the way, and it was an experience I am glad I went through. I, an ordinary staff nurse with no research experience, completed a research study. And believe it or not, I am now involved in a second research study. I keep a list of potential topics, so I am always ready with the next research problem when the urge hits me.

As I move forward with my second research study, I am passing along my best advice to my coinvestigator. These are the things I learned along the way during my initial journey down Research Road.

KNOW (AND USE) YOUR RESOURCES

We had identified for us the resources that were going to make this study possible. We needed and used all of them. It will minimize frustration if you know who your "go to" people are. Our most precious resources were an experienced researcher, a statistician, a librarian, and someone with editorial skills. Our director is doctorally prepared and experienced in research. She guided us along the way and answered what were, I am sure, very basic questions, although they seemed foreign to us. We also were fortunate enough to have the guidance of an internationally renowned nurse researcher who is affiliated with our local university.

Our hospital had retained the services of an outside consultant who became our "numbers guy." We spoke to the statistician at various points on our journey. He helped us to ensure that we were asking the right questions, assisted with creating our data collection spreadsheet, and talked to us about sample size and how the analyses would be done. He also offered suggestions about other potential analyses that could be done that we had not thought of. He was indispensable.

Our medical librarian was another gift. A literature review becomes never-ending. It is perpetual, right up through when the manuscript is with the editors. Just when you think you've hit them all, someone finds another related study. A close working relationship with our librarian meant that she knew the topic of study and always had her eyes open for newly appearing literature.

The editorial skill (of someone else) is invaluable. At times, after looking at a document for too long, we become immune to the most basic grammar mistakes and misspellings. Our editor worked with us from the proposal phase all the way to the final manuscript. Again, another essential tool for a successful journey.

LITERATURE REVIEW

Don't ever assume that your literature review is complete and exhaustive. I found that it never was. Each time I went to "check one last time," I found more related articles, and some were ones that could not be ignored. Even at the point of publication, the editors requested a more updated literature review. We were given the tip of starting a reference list from the beginning, which has paid off in the case of the great article that goes missing. It is also helpful, as you gather articles, to develop some type of key so that articles can be quickly identified as research/not research, useful/not useful. This can be done with simple notations: R (research) and NR (not research), and Y (yes helpful) and N (not helpful).

PROPOSAL

When beginning your proposal, think of the final product, which, according to my director and which I now believe, is the published manuscript. Set up the proposal in a manner that resembles the makings of a journal article. Get all the headings (introduction, research question, literature review, theoretical framework, methodology, intervention, data analysis, and so on) needed for a published article; this becomes your framework for your proposal. Then, as you move toward a final manuscript, it is all right there, and all you have to do is beef it up.

DATA COLLECTION

In the beginning, we thought we had an organized data collection system. In the end, it turned out that it could have been better. I would recommend that your statistician see your data collection tool with some trail data entered. This will give him or her a chance to make sure that you are collecting your data in a way that is optimal for data analysis. For example, in our data collection tool, we used Y or N for responses that required a yes or no answer; if the data were for male or female, we used M or F. We did not know (we were very new researchers) that all data had to be in numbers (e.g., yes = 1, no = 2). As you begin your data collection, have a notebook so that you can list your limitations as you go along. We used little sticky post notes any time we found a limitation that we wanted to include in the study. In the end, they were too hard to keep track of. Listing the limitations from the beginning in an organized fashion will help with the manuscript at the end.

When embarking on a research study, I would recommend that you have the support of your supervisor. When you have the support of key individuals and research is a priority for the hospital, your workload and priorities can be adjusted as needed. One of my concerns when taking on this research study was that my other responsibilities would take priority and I would never get to the research. This did not happen, and my supervisor made sure of this. Establishing a timeline is another effective method of keeping to task and ensuring that things get done. The timeline can be fluid and flexible, but it functions as a good guide to getting things done. And finally, I recommend a coinvestigator. Having someone else to work with is beneficial because not only can you share the workload, but you also have someone else's perspective when it comes time to make decisions. Without a doubt, each investigator will have his or her own strengths and weaknesses, and this can help determine the roles that each person plays.

Reducing Restraint Use in an Acute Care Hospital: Evaluation of a Restraint Reduction Initiative and the Impact on the Fall Rate

Mary Beth Strauss, MS, RN, BC

Purpose: A retrospective research study was conducted in a 200-bed acute care community hospital to examine the effects of a restraint reduction initiative on both the use of restraints and the fall rate among hospitalized adult patients.

Methodology:

Setting and Sample

This research study was conducted in a 200-bed, not-for-profit Massachusetts acute care community hospital. The investigators were staff development specialists. Interrater reliability was established through a 10-chart review. The data collected for this project were drawn from the hospital's five medical-surgical units (118 beds) and one intensive care unit (10 beds). The sample population for this project included all adult medical-surgical patients placed in medical-surgical restraints, as defined by the hospital (**Table 25-1**), between April 1, 2001, and February 28, 2002. Because the fall rates were investigated as well, patients who experienced a fall, as documented in the hospital's incident report, during this time period were also included. Patients were excluded from the data if they were chemically restrained, in behavioral restraints, restrained under the hospital's clinical protocol, or restrained only through the use of side rails.

Intervention

A restraint reduction initiative was instituted in July 2001. This initiative provided hospital systems improvements and an educational program in which 95% of the nursing staff participated.

As part of this program, a multidisciplinary performance improvement team was formed, and its task was to find ways to safely reduce restraint use. Policies and documentation tools were revised and competencies were developed

Table 25-1   Definitions of Restraints

Restraint Category	Definition
Physical Restraint	"Any method of physically restricting a person's freedom of movement or normal access to one's own body" (Winchester Hospital, 2001).
Medical/Surgical Restraint	"Restraint use in response to behavior that prevents active treatment of medical/surgical problems or when the intent is to promote physical recovery or healing" (Winchester Hospital, 2001).
Behavioral Restraint	"Restraint use driven by a behavioral health problem. Limited to emergencies where there is imminent risk of an individual physically harming him/herself or others" (Winchester Hospital, 2001).
Chemical Restraint	"Any medication used to control behavior or to restrict the patient's freedom of movement . . . and is not a standard treatment for the patient's condition" (Winchester Hospital, 2001).
Clinical Protocol	"Restraint use in response to patients attempting to remove therapeutic devices that are essential to medical/surgical healing. Such devices include, but are not limited to, endotracheal tubes, catheters or intravenous lines" (Winchester Hospital, 2001).

Source: Winchester Hospital. (2001). Restraint safety devices, use of. *Patient Care Services Policy & Procedure Manual.* Winchester, MA: Author.

based on current research. Restraint reduction manuals, used as resources for the nurses, were developed for every unit. The team created a diversional activity cart, which was available to all units (**Table 25-2**). This cart was used to provide activities to those patients at risk to be restrained.

The other components of this initiative were largely educational. Registered nurses, licensed practical nurses, clinical associates, and managers and supervisors were required to attend a 1-hour workshop that emphasized regulations regarding restraints, classifications of restraints, and alternatives to restraints. Possible causes of mental confusion and strategies to reduce these

Table 25-2   Diversional Activity Cart

Contents of the Diversional Activity Cart
• Cassette player
• Music tapes and headphones
• Puzzles
• Books and magazines
• Word search/crossword puzzles
• Playing cards
• Socks to match and fold
• Activity board
• Computer keyboard
• Videos
• Knitting supplies

factors were reviewed. Educational posters were designed for the units, and the same education was incorporated into nursing orientation.

Data collection

Data were collected for the 3 months before implementation of the program (April through June 2001), for the 2 months during program implementation (July through August 2001), and for 6 months after implementation (September 2001 through February 2002). Data gathered during the 2 months of program implementation were considered preintervention data. All data were gathered retrospectively by the two investigators. Data collection sources were the daily restraint log, incident report form, patient record, and electronic patient care database. The daily restraint log was used to determine which patients were in restraints during the time period studied. The incident report was used to gather information regarding patients who fell during this time period. Information gathered from the incident report included activity at the time of fall, age of patient who fell, time of fall, and medications taken prior to the fall. The patient record was used to determine length of restraint event, type of restraint, and admitting diagnosis of the patient. The electronic patient care database was used to gather patient demographic data and information regarding length of stay.

A restraint event is measured from the time when an individual is first restrained and ends when the use of restraint ceases, regardless of the number of orders or renewals (Maryland Hospital Association, 2001).

A fall is defined as an "unplanned movement of a patient to the ground or from one plane to another" (Maryland Hospital Association, 2001).

The injury sustained by a patient is classified according to the description of the injury on the hospital's incident report. The injury level ranges from a Level 1 (*no apparent injury*) to a Level 4 (*injury occurred with resulting treatment or intervention required*). The injury level is determined by the individual nurse and/or supervisor completing the document.

Results:

Restraints

There was no significant difference in gender among the restrained patients. **Table 25-3** displays age and length of stay for all patients restrained from April 2001 through February 2002 ($n = 106$) in comparison with all adult medical-surgical patients in the hospital for the same time period. **Table 25-4** illustrates the top four admitting diagnoses for the study group of restrained patients.

Restraint usage was analyzed using the total number of hospital days associated with restraint use and those hospital days associated with no restraint use. Using patient days as a measure, we were able to determine the number of patient days with restraints and without restraints in both the preintervention and postintervention periods. **Table 25-5** shows these data. If the intervention

Table 25-3   **Age and Length of Stay for Restrained Patients versus All Adult Medical-Surgical Patients**

Group	Average Age	Average Length of Stay
Study group	82 years	7.3 days
Hospital group	56.5 years	3.7 days

Note: n = 106

Table 25-4   Admission Diagnoses for Restrained Patients

Ranking	Admitting Diagnosis	Frequency	Percentage
1	Congestive heart failure*	8	7.5%
2	• Pneumonia* • UTI	7 7	6.6% 6.6%
3	Syncope	6	5.7%
4	• Hip fracture* • Acute myocardial infarction* • Volume depletion*	5 5 5	4.7% 4.7% 4.7%

Note: * = top hospital diagnoses.

Table 25-5   Restraint Usage Pre/Postintervention

Patient Days	Preintervention	Postintervention
Patient days without restraints	16,290 days	21,238 days
Patient days with restraints	554 days	232 days

has a positive impact, the ratio of patient days with a restraint to patient days without a restraint would be lower after the intervention than before.

The chi-square test, based on Table 25-5, demonstrates that restraint usage dropped significantly after the initiative (X^2 = 229.1; df = 1; p < .001). Examination of the table indicates that the percent of patient days with restraints in the preintervention period is more than 3 times as large as the percent of patient days with restraints in the postintervention period (1.33% vs. 0.4%).

Figure 25-1 illustrates how the ratio of restraint use dropped over the course of 11 months. This ratio was derived from the number of restraints over the number of patient days for each month and then multiplied by 1,000 to make the resulting ratio a number above 1. The correlation between month and this ratio is significant (r = −.88, p < .001).

Figure 25-1   Restraint Use Ratio by Month

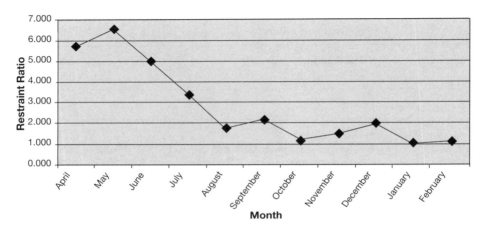

Falls

There was no significant difference between genders for the group of patients who fell. **Table 25-6** illustrates the average age and length of stay for the patients who fell ($n = 123$) as compared with all adult medical-surgical patients during the same time period. The top four diagnoses for patients who fell are listed in **Table 25-7**.

To calculate the intervention's impact on the number of falls, as with restraint use, the number of patient days with falls and the number of patient days without falls for each time period were entered into a 2×2 chi-square table (**Table 25-8**). The findings of this project demonstrate that after the restraint reduction intervention, the fall rate was significantly

Table 25-6   Age and Length of Stay for Patients Who Fell versus All Adult Medical-Surgical Patients

Group	Average Age	Average Length of Stay
Study group	75 years	8.7 days
Hospital group	56.5 years	3.7 days

Table 25-7　Admitting Diagnoses for Patients Who Fell

Ranking	Admitting Diagnosis	Frequency	Percentage
1	Pneumonia*	12	9.8%
2	Volume depletion*	11	8.9%
3	Acute CVA*	8	6.5%
4	• Congestive heart failure* • UTI • Fever	5 5 5	4.1% 4.1% 4.1%

Note: * = top hospital diagnoses.

Table 25-8　Falls Pre/Postintervention

Patient Days	Preintervention	Postintervention
Patient days without falls	16,233 days	21,028 days
Patient days with falls	611 days	442 days

reduced (x^2 = 86.9; df = 1; p < .001 level). Although the decline was not as dramatic for falls, the table indicates that the percent of patient days with falls in the preintervention period is nearly twice as large as the percent of patient days with falls in the postintervention period (3.63% vs. 2.05%).

Figure 25-2 illustrates this reduction in the fall ratio. The fall ratio was calculated from the number of falls over the number of patient days multiplied by 1,000 to produce a number greater than 1.

Restraints and Falls
For patients who were restrained at the time of a fall (n = 20), there was no statistical difference in the injury level when compared with those not restrained at the time of a fall, t (120) = −.953, p = .342.

Conclusion: Restraint use and falls have an economic impact and a physical and emotional impact. It is important for educators to examine the pattern

Figure 25-2   Fall Ratio by Month

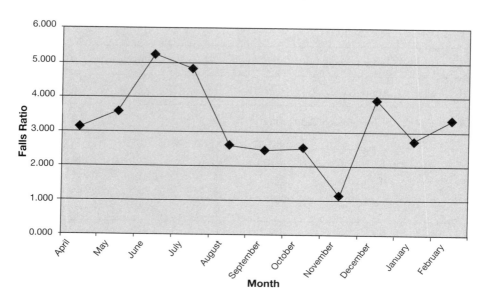

of restraint use in their institutions and provide the necessary education and support to make it possible to safely reduce their use. A restraint reduction initiative must be multifaceted and include both a strong educational component and a reliance on restraint alternatives. Nurses must be able to accurately identify patients at risk for a restraint event or a fall and implement a plan of care to ensure the safest possible environment for that patient.

REFERENCES

Maryland Hospital Association. (2001). *Quality indicator report: Acute care implementation manual.* Elkridge, MD: Author.

Winchester Hospital. (2001). Restraint safety devices, use of. *Patient care services policy & procedure manual.* Winchester, MA: Author.

CHAPTER 26

Bedside Nursing Research: How We Made a Difference!

Janet Brock

I was just minding my own business. I was working on my acute general medicine unit just like I had done for the past 11 years. I was taking care of my patients' needs the best I could according to the "Guidelines and Policies." And I was doing everything the way we always do it because—well—that is the way we have always done it, and besides, it is right here in *the manual*—in black and white. Little did I know that my whole world of black and white and policies and procedures was about to come tumbling down.

This was the day of never turning back. I was approached by our unit's Clinician 4. She explained that she was taking on a new project (which usually means that I am also taking on a new project). She was participating in a new nursing research mentor group. This group's task was to gather a group of nurses who work at the patient's bedside and start a research project. As she was excitedly talking and explaining the whole process, my mind began to wander. It was mostly wondering, *Why is she talking to me about this?* I don't know anything about research. I have an associate's degree in nursing, and nursing research was not part of our curriculum. I can assess my patients, give medications, provide assistance with hydration and elimination, monitor vital signs, and communicate effectively with and about my patients. I am a strong patient advocate and provide excellent customer service to my patients and their families. I maintain professionalism at all times, note subtle changes in my patients' condition, and communicate with the appropriate staff. I change my plan of care to accommodate a critically ill patient until an ICU bed is available, and I complete the 120 pages of documentation to prove that I did everything I was supposed to do and in the way that I am supposed to do it. And now they want to add nursing research to my day? I don't even own a pair of goggles. I haven't used a Petri dish or a microscope in years. Visions of Bunsen burners and flasks with multicolored smoke danced around in my head. And there I was—me—standing over all that smoke with my hair in disarray (OK, my hair usually is in disarray) looking rather pale, like I hadn't seen the light of day for several months. There I was with charts and graphs, lots of chemicals and hazardous materials, and then there was the laugh—the evil laugh of mad women stuck behind closed doors, all in the name of nursing research!

As my mind exhaustedly came back to the Clinician 4, the only thing that could escape from my lips was, "OK, anything for my patients." (You already know that nurses have a hard time saying no.)

We were able to get a significant number of nurses interested in this project. We met weekly and brainstormed about our patient population. What are the main diagnoses of our patients? We had pages and pages of nursing diagnoses, complications, and issues with our patient population. We began to narrow down the number of pages. What are the things that nursing can change? After weeks and weeks of discussion and changing our minds, the issue of central line dressings kept creeping back into the conversations. The dressing that we were using at that time often lost adherence, and dressings were changed more frequently than in our protocol. The need for multiple dressing changes led to an increased risk of infection for the patient, increased nursing time, and an increased cost to the facility. We decided to compare several different types of central line dressings to see which best adhered to the patient's skin. We were looking for the dressing that remained occlusive consistently for the longest period of time.

After 3 months of data collection, we discovered that one dressing type was superior in maintaining adherence. Our research findings were shared with our institution's clinical practice committee, equipment supply committee, professional nursing staff organization, and at the Evidence-Based Best Practice Day. As a result of our research, our institution changed the standard of practice for central venous catheter dressings (CVC). We also presented our research poster at the National Academy of Medical Surgical Nurses Convention in Las Vegas, and our article has been accepted for publication in a peer-reviewed nursing journal.

Imagine, me the nurse, just here minding my own business, standing before the leadership of our institution sharing nursing research findings. Me, the nurse who doesn't own a pair of goggles, has traveled across the country and shared nursing research findings at a national convention in Las Vegas. Me, the nurse just trying to take care of my patients, now researching and discovering the best way to care for my patients. I now understand the meaning of *evidence-based practice* in a way that I never understood it before. It is my responsibility to my patients and my profession to ask, "Why do we do this, and what is the evidence behind the way we are doing it?" Those black and white books on the shelf are no longer just black and white books sitting on the shelf; they are the living evidence of a nurse's desire to bring evidence-based practice to the bedside. The books are a result of research by a nurse just like me, and hopefully you, who have had your eyes and mind opened by an idea that could possibly make a difference in patients' outcomes and in the daily life of another nurse.

I think all nurses are always wondering, *Why do we do this, and wouldn't that make more sense?* It is the nurse providing the direct care to the patient who would best know what the problems and barriers to patient care are. Doesn't it just make sense that the nurse providing the direct care be the nurse asking the questions and finding the answers? Obviously, nursing research has very little to do with goggles, flasks, and Petri dishes. Nursing research occurs when the nurse does the right thing by providing patient care using the scientific evidence!

My advice to other nurses is: Don't do things just because that is what has always been done. Ask questions and search for the answers. If you can't find evidence-based research for your practice, question it and then just do the research yourself. If research is new to you, then find a mentor and tackle the questions. Don't be afraid of what you may find. You may make a difference in the quality of your patient's care or outcomes. You may make a difference in your peers' daily work life. You may make changes that affect your whole institution. Who knows, you might be writing in one of those black and white books one day (*the manual*)!

Acknowledgment: I would like to acknowledge the University of Virginia's Professional Nursing Staff Organization for supporting, encouraging, and promoting nursing research. I am also thankful for the guidance and teaching of Suzi Burns, the "research guru." Thanks to Barb Trotter for always pushing me to the limits and always finding something to occupy my time, and laughing with me along the way. All our research was made possible by our supportive managers Jodean Chisholm and Juanita Day, and the nurses of 3 West and 3 Central. This is our story.

Central Venous Catheter Dressings: Tape/Gauze versus Transparent Dressing

Janet Brock, ADN, RN

Central venous catheters (CVCs) are an integral component of the care of the acutely ill patient. In comparison with peripheral catheters, CVCs are used for long-term venous access. It is essential that CVC dressings remain intact. At our institution, numerous methods for assuring proper securement of the CVC were commonly used. These included tape/gauze dressing, transparent dressing, or a combination of the two.

Purpose: The purpose of our study was to compare three different CVC dressing methods to assess the occlusiveness/adherence.

Design: The study was a convenience sample of patients with CVCs on two adult acute care units.

Methods: Subjects were randomly assigned to three CVC dressing methods:

- The "central line kit," a prepackaged kit. This included 2×2 gauze and Durapore tape.
- The Tegaderm transparent dressing (10×12 cm) and 2×2 gauze. This was our standard dressing method.
- SorbaView 2000 transparent dressing.

All three methods used a ChloraPrep (chlorhexidine gluconate 2%) skin preparation.

Results: The transparent dressing, SorbaView, proved to be statistically significant in dressing adherence as compared with the tape/gauze dressing. This study helped establish a standard for the CVC dressings in our health system.

Conclusion: The routine dressing change standard of M, W, F changed for our health system to once a week, in accordance with CDC guidelines. Therefore, there is the potential for a significant cost savings in terms of supplies and nursing time. Because of our findings, we were able to present our research at our institution's Evidence-Based Practice Day. Subsequently, we presented our findings at a national medical-surgical nursing conference, and our article has been accepted for publication in *American Nurse Today*.

CHAPTER 27

In the Beginning:
My Initiation into Research

Cheryl G. Newmark

I have to be honest; I never really thought much about the research process! It was always something that someone else initiated. I would read about studies in my nursing journals every month but was never really moved by any of them. They seemed to be full of terms and statistical analysis information that I found very confusing! I would always feel lost somewhere in the middle of the study.

In 2002, I attended my first New Jersey Emergency Nurses Association (ENA) Emergency Care Conference in Atlantic City. There in the registration area was a big board asking for volunteers for different committees for ENA. I noticed that one of the areas listed was for volunteers for a boating and recreational injury research study that would be started in conjunction with the United States Coast Guard and ENA. Because my husband and I owned a boat and enjoyed boating and fishing, I thought this might be interesting. The purpose of that study was to look for reasons that so many boating and recreational vehicle injuries were occurring in America's waterways. I signed up and was very surprised to get a letter from the ENA thanking me for volunteering and informing me that I would hear from the research department shortly. I was sent to Washington DC to attend a seminar about the study and learned so much about the research process. At that point, I was hooked! That study ran for 4 years. As the site coordinator for the project, it was my responsibility to pick a research team and in-service them about the study itself and the research process. I used this opportunity to learn about and get to know my hospital's institutional review board (IRB) and types of consents, as well as how to formulate an abstract and how to tabulate the information from the teaching tool. I learned about ICD-9 codes and in-serviced a new team of investigators for each year of the study.

The particular study that I am working on at the present time came about while I was in the triage area in the emergency department (ED). I would greet patients in triage and ask them about allergies and if they took any medications on a daily basis. I was amazed and somewhat disheartened to see that many of the patients who presented to me in triage had no idea of certain aspects of their medications. Some would tell me the name of the drug they were taking but could not tell me why they were taking it. Others could tell me that they had, for example, high cholesterol and took a blue pill but did not know the name of the pill. Many gave the answer that their physician just told them to take the medication. Still others would tell me that they were not sure when they were supposed to take the medication and that they took it whenever they remembered. I found this to be very frustrating, and I seemed to hear it over and over again. I went to my manager and discussed this problem with her. I told her I would love to do a research study on this problem. After she gave me her blessing and support, I set out to find someone who could help me begin my own research study. I was very excited at the prospect of starting my own study!

I had the good fortune of meeting a nurse researcher at a nursing education council meeting. She listened to my idea for the study and jumped in with both feet! She was totally supportive and encouraged me to start immediately.

We began by doing a literature review of patients and their medications. From there, we constructed a consent form for the patients to sign and sent it through to the hospital IRB. We then began putting together the paperwork that would be necessary for this study. We looked at both inclusion and exclusion criteria and developed a tool by which we could keep a record of patients' progress with the study. While I was at another ENA conference in San Antonio, I came across a medication card that would be the perfect tool for my study: a patient reminder of his or her medications.

In July 2007, I officially started to solicit patients for my study as they came into the triage area in the ED. I explained the study and why I felt that it was an important study to do. I was delighted to see a positive response from patients. Many of them agreed and were honest in admitting that they did not remember what the names of their medications were, when to take them, and why they were taking them. Some would just say that their doctors told them to take it but did not get into specifics about the medications themselves.

I have just signed my last patient into the study. It has taken me 5 months to obtain all the patients I need for the study. Now it is time to start the next and final phase. I have received so much praise from my peers and nursing personnel in the hospital when they hear about my study. It makes me proud to know that I was able to launch my own study, which came about from a problem that I had recognized. I have learned so much by being given that first opportunity to join in a research study. It opened up another realm of nursing in which I had no previous knowledge.

My advice to others who may be afraid to join in or start a study of their own is to sit in on a nursing research committee at their place of employment.

Read some studies on a topic that you may be interested in. If you have an idea for a study, do not think that it is a useless idea. Present it to your manager or the head of nursing research; they are always interested in ideas for studies. I look at my study as a positive extension of my nursing career. I am currently a graduate student at Thomas Edison State College, going for my MSN in nursing education. My ultimate goal is to become a nursing instructor so I can give something back to this wonderful profession that I have been a part of for 32 years. I want to teach our nurses of tomorrow.

Acknowledgment: I would like to thank so many people for helping me and believing in me as I begin my research journey. Thank you to my mentor, Sue Fowler, PhD, RN, for her guidance and wealth of knowledge of nursing research. I could not have done this project without her patience and commitment, to believe in this study and help me realize that I actually had the potential to begin a study of my own.

Thank you to my nurse manager in the emergency department, Carol Jones, MSN, RN, APN, for giving me the courage and the opportunity to begin this research study. She gave me positive feedback and the motivation to believe in myself and my study. I would like to thank the staff in the ED for their assistance with the study as well as their constant support.

Finally, a big thank you to my husband, Michael, and my sons, Eric and Neal. My family has been a constant source of support to me, and without their encouragement, I would not be where I am today.

Patient Knowledge of Medications in the ED

Cheryl G. Newmark, BSN, RN

Purpose: To ascertain if the use of a medication card to patients will increase their knowledge of medications and communication with their healthcare provider.

Problem: Patients are not able to articulate their prescribed medications, including names, dosages, purpose, schedule, and/or food–drug interactions. Their lack of awareness puts them at risk for drug interactions, duplicate medications, and absence of medications. Strategies need to assist patients to be empowered about their medication practices at home.

Design: Descriptive survey and interventional design

Methodology: Convenience sampling ($N = 20$). Subject enrolled if cognitively alert, English-speaking middle-aged adults (30–70 years of age) who have been prescribed four or more medications who present to the emergency department (ED) and are discharged home from ED.

Procedure: Within 3 days of enrollment, subjects receive a letter via mail along with a medication card and medication sheets. Subjects are called, using a script, 10 days after their ED visit to inquire about completion of the medication card and/ or knowledge of medications. A second phone call is made to those subjects who lack the understanding of how to complete the medication card. A letter is sent to all patients' healthcare providers, informing them of the subject's participation in study, knowledge of medications, and medication card. The letter also suggests that healthcare providers make a copy of the patient's medication card at the next visit and to make a concerted effort to keep the card updated with any new medications. At 4 months after study initiation, a call will be placed to the healthcare providers of study patients to inquire about their patient's use of medication cards during office visits.

Results: At this time, all 20 study participants have been sent the study package materials and have been contacted by the principal investigator. Final results and conclusions are pending.

CHAPTER 28

My Nursing Research Path

Alison Chappell

As with most new nurses, my exposure to nursing research began with research classes as a student. However, as a new nurse, my interest in research was sparked by my nursing manager. She asked me to represent our general medical unit on the Georgetown University Hospital-based Performance Improvement and Research Council, a division of shared governance. During my first research council meeting (actually maybe even for the first 6 months), I was very quiet and shy and completely unsure of what my role would be within this council and with nursing research. I have a degree in biology, and I have had many experiences with scientific research as an undergraduate student, but nursing research, in my mind, was not quite as clearly delineated as biological research. As a member of this Georgetown University Hospital Nursing Research Council, I had the opportunity to assist as a coinvestigator on a research project entitled Peripheral Vascular Access Acquisition Using the Transvenous Illuminator. During this research process, I learned that I was intimidated by the institutional review board (IRB). I suspect that many new nurses are as well. Yet as a coinvestigator, I had the ability to assist with the research proposal process and obtain a better understanding of the research process. This initial research project was a great learning experience. Prior to being a coinvestigator for a study, my nurse manager and nurse educator encouraged me to lead a performance improvement project, Effectiveness of Nursing Interventions in the Prevention of Hospital-Acquired Urinary Tract Infections. I had the opportunity to present this project at the National Academy of Medical Surgical Nurses conference in September 2006. Performance improvement projects are a wonderful way to begin your quest toward nursing research.

Later, I became the cochair of the Performance Improvement and Research Council. As a cochair, I had a great desire to lead a hospital-wide nursing research project. Initially, I was unsure of the topic. Through personal and professional situations, end-of-life care became a research interest of mine. I was very involved in the dying process of my grandmother. From my grandmother's passing, I learned that those facing death and their families deserve respect and special care that can be enhanced by properly trained healthcare professionals. The following tells of a work experience concerning one of my more memorable patient care situations involving end-of-life care. This situation profoundly affected me and helped me to realize the need for nurses in the hospital setting to be trained in end-of-life care.

Ms. M, a general medicine patient, was completely nonverbal. She was recently admitted to the hospital from a nursing home and ordered to receive comfort care only. On the second or third day of caring for Ms. M, I realized that she had no visitors or calls concerning her clinical status. She was dying all alone, and I was concerned that I could not give her the attention she needed and deserved. On this particular afternoon, I was surprised to receive a phone call from the chaplain at an area prison. The reason for the call became clear when the chaplain placed Ms. M's son on the telephone. I was unable to convey much concerning his mother's condition to the son because of privacy regulations. Yet I wanted him to have the chance to say goodbye to his mother to aid him in coping with her death and to help her have a more peaceful transition. Ms. M's son had no idea about the severity of her illness, and he was estranged from his sister and brother. During the conversation, he emphasized his realization that he would never see his mother again because of the actions that led to his prison sentence. Although Ms. M was completely nonverbal, I felt that it was necessary for her son to speak to her. I realize the importance of closure in the dying process to both the dying individual and his or her loved ones. He asked me if she was able to speak to him. I told Ms. M's son that she would probably not be able to speak but that I would place the phone by her ear so that she could hear his words. I transferred the phone call to her hospital room. Then, I donned an isolation gown as a Georgetown nursing student watched from the door. I could hear Ms. M's son's words as he spoke to his mother on the telephone. He told her numerous times how much he loved her. He began to sob, and tears began to roll down my face as well. Ms. M's son apologized for his actions, asked for her forgiveness, and told her how much he missed her. He told her what a wonderful woman and mother she had been. During the conversation, Ms. M blinked her eyes, and she seemed to hear his voice. Somehow I know that she was able to comprehend her son's words. I feel that they were both addressing unresolved issues prior to her death. I was able to reassure Ms. M's son that I believed his mother heard him and understood his message. After exiting the room, I talked with the nursing student about the importance of the nurse's role during the dying process. Our actions as nurses, no matter the magnitude, can benefit our patients. I hope that my actions and our conversation will influence her future practice with death and dying. One day after this incident, I returned to the hospital and learned that Ms. M had indeed died the day after this conversation occurred. In some inexplicable way, I feel that my efforts made Ms. M's death easier for both Ms. M and her son.

This incident prompted me to learn more about death and dying and ignited my interest in end-of-life research. I saw the pivotal role that nurses play while providing comfort during end-of-life situations for the patient and the patient's loved ones. I realized that I lacked education on this topic and needed to know more to be as effective a caregiver as possible. With the assistance of coinvestigators and research consultants, including a statistician, my road to research has led to the survey, "End-of-Life Care: Nurses' Beliefs of the Current Care at Georgetown University Hospital." Over 400 nurses participated in this survey. I feel that the success of this project was due to the support and assistance of upper management at Georgetown University Hospital, including the chief nursing officer, Dr. Joyce E. Johnson. I am still amazed by the number of nurses who participated in this research! With the assistance of the Davis Grant for funding, our research team was able to host an end-of-life training session, specifically the curriculum of the End of Life Nursing Consortium (ELNEC) SuperCore course, as a follow-up to the study. This project is still in the research phase, and a follow-up study will be conducted to determine the effectiveness of the educational intervention. Based on my experience with nursing research, I suggest that nurses new to research create a good research team (including consultants and statisticians) and get support from management at their institution. The road to research has many paths, but I hope that mine has encouraged in you the belief that nursing research is fundamental to evolving, growing, and excelling in nursing care.

Acknowledgment: Thanks to Judi Bailey, BSN, RN, nurse manager, and Rayma Skinner, PhD, RN, BSN, nurse educator, for sparking my interest in nursing research. And thanks to Maureen McLaughlin, PhD, RN, and Gail Thurkauf, MSN, RN, for their constant support and guidance through the research process.

End-of-Life Care: Nurses' Beliefs of the Current Care at Georgetown University Hospital, Washington, DC

Alison Chappell, BSN, RN, CMSRN

Purpose: The purpose of this study was to assess the quality of end-of-life care as reported by Georgetown University Hospital registered nurses.

Design: This institutional review board-approved study used a nonexperimental, exploratory survey design. The Quality Care at the End of Life Survey, a 33-item instrument, was used to assess registered nurses' beliefs about the physical, psychological, social, spiritual, cultural, and ethical aspects of end-of-life care.

Methods: Following individual nursing unit promotion of this study, an electronic version of the survey was offered on nursing unit computers to all staff nurses in both inpatient and outpatient settings for a period of 3 weeks. A total of 427 nurses participated in the survey.

Results: With a response rate of 40%, results indicated that 89% of the nurses believe that end-of-life education is a very important component in their basic nursing education. Yet, 52% of the nurses had never received any training on end-of-life care. In 6 months prior to the survey date, 42% of nurses had been involved in one to three end-of-life-care situations. The survey results had a mean of 4.07 for all questions answered based on a 7-point Likert scale.

Conclusions: Only moderate results on each of the aspects of end-of-life care and more than 52% of nurses reporting that they had never received any training justified the need for an educational intervention. An ELNEC Super-Core course was provided to approximately 150 nurses on April 19, 2008. During this 8-hour course, experts on end-of-life care spoke about the eight SuperCore modules: palliative care nursing; pain management; communication; cultural considerations; ethical issues; loss, grief, and bereavement issues; symptom management; and final hours. Further research is necessary to determine the effectiveness of the educational intervention.

(August 2007)

CHAPTER 29

The Reluctant Researchers

Judith Cavanaugh and Julie A. Kenney

The first reluctant researcher, Judi, has been out of graduate school since 1987. Memories of her school research project with neonatal nurses, which was not her area of clinical expertise, were less than palatable. The other reluctant researcher, Julie, is currently in graduate school and therefore much more open to the idea of a research project because of the inevitability of having to do one for school. It helped matters immensely that her focus is healthcare informatics, and our research project focuses on documentation in the electronic health record (EHR).

How did we get here, you ask? We had a brilliant idea for our RN orientation program, which meant writing a proposal for a capital expenditure for 30 laptop computers. The proposal we wrote was accepted, the laptop computers were purchased, and we, of course, had to justify the expenditure. And so the story begins. Because we are part of a healthcare system with multiple sites, the rollout of our EHR as a system initiative has been progressive and labor intensive. Therefore, the acceptance and comfort levels have varied. Our goal was to make the orientation process more interactive. Incorporating the teaching of the EHR in conjunction with the didactic components was an opportune way to achieve this goal. We are achieving more hands-on exposure to the EHR system, which we propose will increase accuracy of documentation and enhance associate comfort levels.

The data collection phase began in July 2007 and ended in April 2008. Our feelings about the project have become less antagonistic in light of the positive reaction that the new associates have shown for the new teaching method. It has also been rewarding for us to see the improvement in documentation accuracy that is due to additional exposure to the EHR during the orientation process. Reports show that the new associates exhibit a greater ease of navigation during the separate EHR class, which pulls everything together using a hands-on teaching method and case studies to enhance the learning experience.

Our nurse researcher approached us about initiating the research project and presenting a poster at a local conference. We have discovered that being involved in nursing research is like an octopus with its many tentacles. Our involvement in various presentations, potential publication efforts, and Julie's comprehensive exam for graduate school generated input from many colleagues and professors. Not only are we living through the research experience, but we are also actually finding the research experience, with its many tentacles, quite interesting. Our advice is to approach the research process with an open mind and with the knowledge that the possibilities for additional exposure related to the activity will be ongoing, if not endless. The best thing we can say is that we have grown throughout this experience, albeit reluctantly, with one another to buffer the storm and with the constant support we received from our nurse researcher.

Acknowledgment: We would like to thank our nurse researcher, Dr. Cheryl Lefavier. She made our research journey easy and enjoyable. We would never have done this without her. We would also like to thank our manager, Debbie O'Connell, for listening to our ideas and providing the equipment and support that we needed to carry out this research project.

Teaching Electronic Documentation: A Comparison of Two Methods

Julie A. Kenney, BSN, RNC, CMSN; and Judith Cavanaugh, MSN, RN-BC

Purpose: The purposes of this study were (1) to determine the difference in knowledge between nurse orientees who were taught skills using computer-based interactive electronic health record (EHR) documentation education, and traditional didactic training with visual presentation, measured by the accuracy of electronic chart documentation, and (2) to determine which teaching method is preferred by nurse orientees.

Design: This quasi-experimental study explored the effects of using electronic documentation during orientation as compared with traditional didactic course lecture.

Methods: All newly employed nurses who completed the orientation coursework participated in the study. The change in instruction technique was incorporated into the orientation program for all nurse orientees. The purpose of the study was disclosed prior to the completion of the documentation case studies. One topic in nurse orientation, IV therapy, was used to evaluate the nurses' understanding and accuracy of documenting in the EHR.

Cohort groups of nurse orientees were organized by the type of method used to teach IV therapy. The control group was taught by the traditional didactic lecture method and demonstration of electronic documentation. The experimental group was taught using a computer-based training module and hands-on practice in conjunction with the computer documentation demonstration. The total sample in each group was to be a minimum of 60 participants.

Understanding of the material was evaluated using a case study that the nurses then documented using the appropriate screens and pathways in the EHR. In addition, all participants were asked to complete an evaluation that included preference questions. Demographic information collected included age, computer use history, and educational level. This demographic information sheet is routinely completed during nurse orientation. Data were analyzed using chi-square and analysis of variance testing.

Results: The sample included 90 subjects in the control group and 106 subjects in the experimental group. Demographically, the groups were similar in age, type of nursing degree, self-rating of computer skills, and self-rating of typing skills. The groups were statistically different ($p = 0.03$) in that the experimental group (32%) had a higher percentage of nurses with more than 1 year of experience than did the control group (23%).

When case study documentation accuracy was analyzed, there was no statistical difference found between groups. Within-group comparisons showed that those in the experimental group who were younger, who had BSN degrees, or who had been exposed to computer documentation did significantly better ($p < 0.05$) when completing the case studies. Younger nurses enrolled in the control group entered a significant number ($p = 0.009$) of correct case study answers, but degree and prior computer documentation experience did not affect the number of correct answers. For all subjects, case study correct responses showed either zero correct or all correct regardless of teaching method. When it came to teaching method satisfaction, the experimental group did have a slightly higher percentage (47.9% vs. 44.6%) of subjects who responded *strongly agree* to question of whether the IV therapy education was adequate to meet their needs. However, there was no statistical difference between groups ($p = 0.228$).

Conclusions: The results suggest that new nurse hires will learn EHR documentation regardless of the teaching methodology, but older nurses may require additional assistance. It may be beneficial for hospitals to implement a computer skills assessment upon hire to assess the need for additional assistance. Hospitals can then enroll these nurses in classes to improve their comfort with computers and with computer documentation.

(2007–2008)

CHAPTER 30

Empowered by Research

Mildred O'Meara-Lett

I had told the director of the Inova Loudoun Hospital (ILH) research council that when a fellow staff nurse asked me to join the research council, I was terrified. She looked at me slightly confused, and with good reason; research was her world, and she understood it very well. I looked at her and said "very," and then reassured her that I wasn't terrified anymore. In fact, I was downright empowered. As an old intensive care unit (ICU) nurse, I was just learning how nurses could make change through doing their own research.

I used to envision research only being done at very large, imposing hospitals and headed by people with at least two PhDs. Now I know that "evidence-based practice" can be started by any bedside nurse who asks the question, *Why?*

It started approximately two years ago. I was asked by an ICU nurse colleague to help her gather data for a study on ventilator-associated pneumonia (VAP) that was being conducted in our ICU. At the time, she was one of our ICU nurses and also the First Research Intern with ILH's research council. Her study was comparing the cost-effectiveness of two endotracheal tubes (ETT) by evaluating VAP rates.

This same colleague broke the news that I would also need to join the research council. I figured I could just sit and hide behind her at these meetings, but it didn't work out quite that way.

First, I had to complete a self-study module from the National Institutes of Health (NIH) on human participants protection, which taught me about some historical events and current issues that affect research today. As I took multiple in-services offered by the research council to hospital staff and was encouraged by the other members of the research council, I became less and less terrified.

Now I no longer sit behind my colleagues. I'm still impressed by the skills and knowledge of the staff who do research at ILH and wish that more nurses knew what power lies at their bedside fingertips.

Acknowledgment: I'd like to acknowledge Karen Gabel Speroni, PhD, RN, the director and the driving force behind Inova Loudoun Hospital's research council, as well as Lisa Dugan, MSN, RN, CNA, BC; Marissa Putnam, MSN, RN, CNA, BC; and Joy Lucas, MSN, RN, CCRN, who, as nurse leaders, encourage their nurses to reach for the highest standards in nursing.

Cost-Effectiveness of Two Endotracheal Tube Types in the Reduction of Ventilator-Associated Pneumonia

Joy Lucas, MSN, RN, CCRN; Karen Gabel Speroni, PhD, RN; Marissa Putman, MSN, RN, CNA, BC; Lisa Dugan, MSN, RN, CNA, BC; Mildred O'Meara-Lett, BS, RN, CCRN; and Marlon G. Daniel, MPH, MHA

Purpose: This study is a comparison of ventilator-associated pneumonia (VAP) rates in patients with standard endotracheal tubes (S-ETT) versus endotracheal tubes with continuous subglottic suctioning (CSS-ETT). The study hypothesis is that the more expensive CSS-ETT will result in a lower VAP rate and will thus be cost-effective.

Design: Prospective two-group comparison of S-ETTs versus CSS-ETTs in intubated patients evaluating incidence of VAP and associated VAP charges.

Methods: Data were collected on 154 patients 18 years or older in one of the following two groups: 77 with the S-ETT, and 77 with CSS-ETT. Patients were excluded if ventilated via tracheostomy or if intubation was less than 48 hours. Data were collected beginning 48 hours after intubation until 48 hours after extubation, discharge, or death. The following date categories were included: demographics, VAP risk factors, intubation, concomitant medications, enteral tube feedings, subglottic suction port clotting, extubation, and reintubation.

Results: There was one case (1.3%) of VAP in the S-ETT group and no cases (0%) if VAP in the CSS-ETT group. Average intubation days for the S-ETT and CSS-ETT group were 5.46 and 7.91 ($p = 0.0173$), respectively. Average ICU days were 9.43 and 11.31 ($p = 0.1047$), respectively. Demographics were comparable between the groups, but the difference in APACHE II scores was statistically significant ($p = 0.0005$), with the S-ETT group being higher. The cost of the endotracheal tubes was \$1.62 (S-ETT) versus \$13.05 (CSS-ETT). Charges for the VAP case were as follows: hospital days = \$68,938.80; ventilator days = \$58,516.22; charges after VAP diagnosis = \$10,422.50.

Conclusions: If a CSS-ETT had been used on all 154 patients, the cost would have been $2,009.70, versus the cost of treating the one VAP in the S-ETT group, $10,422.50. If the CSS-ETT had been used on all patients and the incidence of VAP avoided, the savings would have been $8,412.80. Therefore, it is cost-effective to use the CSS-ETT based on the incidence of VAP rates for the 154 patients in this study.

CHAPTER 31

Never Underestimate the Power of a Nurse!

Laura Reilly

I started my journey into patient quality outcomes and nursing research when my triplets (yes, that's right—triplets!) were two years old. I was a staff nurse in the ICU, and the 12-hour shift requirements were becoming more and more difficult. The desperate phone calls from my husband (who was home alone taking care of three babies while I was at work) were getting more and more despondent. A position became available in the intensive care unit (ICU) for a database coordinator, which required managing a critical care database that tracked ICU patient outcomes. This position would allow me more flexible hours, and it was becoming apparent that this was necessary for my family. I needed to take advantage of the opportunity. I barely knew how to turn on a computer, and I didn't know much about research. What I did know was how important it was to be able to measure what we did so that we knew whether it was working. When I first became interested in conducting research, my biggest concern was how much we, as nurses, underestimated what we could accomplish—how much we, as nurses, did not recognize our own power and abilities. This new role gave me the tools I needed to bring my practice to another level. It required me to take a good look at the validity of our current clinical practice patterns. Where's the evidence? Why are we doing it this way? Is there a better way that will achieve more optimal outcomes?

I think I was open to research because I tend to be someone who enjoys a challenge and welcomes change. I wasn't afraid of research, but I was surrounded by people who were. In the early stages of my research experience, it was very difficult to find anyone who could guide me. Then the Magnet requirements came to my rescue! Our organization has strong nursing leadership and a chief nursing officer dedicated to the "forces of magnetism." A culture of nursing research started to evolve. At first, I really didn't think that most nurses believed that we had the knowledge and the power to really create change. Yet, we were able to affect outcomes in nursing practice that would reach an international level.

Our research study started as a quality improvement initiative that was endorsed by the ICU nurse manager. Our organization supports the Six Sigma quality improvement process, and I was selected to lead a project that would decrease infections in our ICU. Once the initial project was developed, I soon realized that it had evolved into a nursing research project. Off to the institutional review board (IRB) we went.

We completed the study and achieved outstanding results. Everyone was very excited—staff nurses, administration, intensivists, nephrologists, infectious disease physicians, the quality outcomes department staff, and many others who were an integral part of the team. The nurses were inspired when they found out that their hard work paid off! I think the greatest gratification came in knowing that we really made a difference in patient care. Many times, nurses don't know if what they do really improves the outcomes for the patient. By systematically measuring our interventions, we can be sure with high probability (or statistical significance) that the outcome is due to the interventions implemented.

If I can do research, you can too. When I started my journey, I hadn't yet completed my baccalaureate degree. My "love affair" with nursing research and my desire to improve patient outcomes has led me to realize the importance of an advanced degree. I recently graduated with an MSN, and it has provided me with even more of the tools needed to be a successful nurse leader.

The best approach to nursing research is to ask yourself a practice question that you would like to investigate. Once you have a question, read the literature, look for an answer, and find a way to measure it. Start small, but think big, and no matter what, don't give up! Break through the barriers, believe in what you're doing, and believe in yourself. I guarantee it will be worthwhile. And never, ever underestimate the power of a nurse!

The following research project resulted in several poster and podium presentations and an article in a peer-reviewed journal, and it was the winner of the 2005 Innovations in Clinical Excellence Evidence-Based Practice Award sponsored by Sigma Theta Tau and *Nursing Spectrum*. I continue to receive inquiries regarding this project from organizations across the country, as well as international requests, including a university hospital in Italy!

Acknowledgment: I would like to acknowledge the support of the ICU nurse manager, Denise Fochesto, MSN, RN, CCRN, APN-C, and the chief nursing officer, Trish O'Keefe, MSN, RN, CAN, for their dedication to nursing excellence through ongoing Magnet achievements. I would especially like to thank the IRB manager, Paula Bistak, RN, who guided me through the IRB application process and encouraged me to seek the guidance I needed to succeed in nursing research.

Decreasing Foley Catheter Device Days in an ICU: A Six Sigma Approach

Laura Reilly, MSN, CCRN, CNRN

Purpose: Indwelling urinary catheters can lead to many complications, most commonly urinary tract infections (UTIs). Decreasing Foley catheter device days (DDs) will lead to a decrease in UTIs.

Design: This was a quasi-experimental prospective interventional study with a retrospective control.

Methods: A collaborative approach with Six Sigma techniques was used.

A DD began upon admission to the ICU with a catheter or one placed in ICU. A DD ended when discharged from ICU with the Foley catheter or the catheter was discontinued in ICU. A total of 124 patient charts (95% confident sample size) were reviewed retrospectively using a data collection tool that was tested for reliability and reproducibility. The preintervention mean was 4.72 ($n = 124$), and the preintervention standard deviation was 7.67 ($n = 124$). Education for ICU staff included complications associated with prolonged catheterization, a decision-making algorithm, and criteria-based guidelines for Foley catheter use. A daily checklist was completed by the nurses for every patient with a Foley catheter. If the patient did not meet the criteria, the physician was contacted for an order to remove the catheter.

Results: 53 patient charts (95% confident sample size) were reviewed postintervention, mean DD = 2.98 ($n = 83$). A two-sample t test determined a statistically significant change in the means ($p = .03$). The postintervention standard deviation was 3.17 ($n = 83$). A test for equal variances determined a change in standard deviations with 94% confidence ($p = .06$).

Conclusion: Critical care nurses play a vital role in reducing prolonged catheterizations that can lead to UTIs in the critically ill patient. Nursing practice should include preventive standards that can lead to improved patient outcomes.

CHAPTER 32

How Families Pushed Me to the Brink—of Research, That Is!

Sherry (Sharon) Ninni

If you had told me a few years ago that I would be doing research *and* liking it, I would have laughed. Research, to me, was something that was only done by PhDs. I thought it was difficult to read and understand, not to mention boring. It was akin to learning a foreign language. The way I became involved in research is as follows: I work in a critical care area. We had recently changed our visiting hours to allow families to spend more time with their loved ones. This was done because we realized the important role that families play in improved outcomes and satisfaction of patients in the intensive care unit (ICU). An unexpected problem developed: Controlling the flow of families and providing needed support while also caring for their critically ill loved ones was difficult to accomplish. Coming from a large, close-knit family, I could relate to their need to be close to their loved ones and receive information. However, caring for the critically ill patient is the nurse's first priority. How can we provide families with the support they need?

Being a 40-something-year-old, I was initially computer illiterate; I wasn't quite sure where to begin. I learned how to perform an OVID search and was amazed at the results. The fact that I could access and peruse multiple journal abstracts and articles in such a short time frame was marvelous. Critical care family needs are well documented in the literature. I had a wealth of information at my fingertips. A valid and reliable survey that addressed critical care family satisfaction was located. Permission to use the survey was obtained, and we started to send it to all of our patients' families. We also surveyed the nurses. Their results supported the liberal visiting hours but suggested that more assistance was needed to help our families. The use of hospital volunteers was recommended to provide information, direction, and comfort to our families. After collaborating with the manager of the volunteer department, it was decided that the volunteer services program would be implemented.

It was suggested that we do a study to see if the use of the volunteers had an effect on nurse and family satisfaction levels. This is the point at which I became involved in the nursing research committee. To do a study, I had to get a review and approval from our nursing research committee (NRC) and our institutional review board. Going to these meetings opened my eyes to all the research being done in my organization. I became very interested in research and in using the best evidence to provide care for my patients. I joined the evidence-based practice subcommittee of our NRC; I now chair this important subcommittee.

My feelings about research have made a 180-degree turn. I love to read about evidence that supports nursing practice. How can you not want to provide care that results in the best outcomes for your patients? To see statistical evidence that an intervention makes a difference is exciting. I have learned to look for both statistical and clinical significance. Learning how to critically appraise or critique studies has made me cognizant of the fact that you can't believe everything you read. Truly understanding the meaning of statistical terms is enlightening. Look for the "level of evidence" of research studies, the best being randomized controlled studies, and the least being expert opinion.

Advice I can offer is to always question your practice—Why are you doing it this way? Is there another way it can be done that would produce better patient outcomes? What if we did this instead?—and then search for the evidence to support what you are doing or what you want to try. Don't accept "because that's the way we have always done it" as an answer. Many libraries offer classes or have tutorials that provide instruction on how to perform a database search. Don't be frustrated if you can't find the information you are looking for. Nursing research is relatively new, and finding the data to support your plan may be difficult. If you can't find the answers, consider doing a study of your own. Although research can be time consuming, it is fun, and you can contribute to the body of knowledge by doing research in areas in which it has not been done. If there is a lot of information on your topic, look for a meta-analysis, which is a summary of all the available evidence or research articles related to your topic. Develop your questions using the PICO (patient/problem/population, intervention, comparison, and outcome) format to make it easier to find answers. Use key words when doing your search to help you find the information you are looking for. Join or start a journal club in your area. Pick an interesting article that applies to your area of specialty and compare it with how you currently practice. Broaden your horizons by joining a hospital- or organization-based research committee. The more you look at articles, the easier understanding the terminology will become. Look up any statistical terms that you are unfamiliar with. Believe me, there is nothing to be afraid of—it's not as bad as you think!

Acknowledgment: The author acknowledges Susan B. Fowler, PhD, MMH, clinical nurse researcher, for her support and assistance.

The Effects of a Volunteer Services Program on Family Satisfaction and Nurse Satisfaction in a Medical/Surgical/Trauma ICU

Sherry (Sharon) Ninni, BSN, RN, CCRN

Purpose: The purpose of the volunteer services program (VSP) is to provide support, guidance, and information to family members of critically ill patients. The care of the family is a vital component in obtaining optimal patient outcomes and improving satisfaction levels. Critical care family needs are significant and well documented. This study will evaluate the effect of the program on family and nurse satisfaction in an intensive care unit (ICU). This effect will be measured using a proven valid and reliable survey tool.

Design: This is a pre- and postimplementation study based on survey results.

Methods: Interested volunteers were carefully selected and provided with a thorough orientation. Volunteers were used during our "quiet time," which provided scheduled rest periods for the nurses, and at change of shift, when nurses provided reports to other nurses taking over the care of their patients. They were stationed at the entrance to the ICU to answer questions, provide support and guidance, and facilitate communication. A survey was distributed to all ICU families pre- and postimplementation of the VSP. Nurse satisfaction with the VSP will be determined using analysis of a pre- and post-VSP survey.

Results: An analysis of the results of the survey returns pre- and postimplementation of the VSP demonstrated a significant improvement in overall satisfaction levels ($p = .03$). The nursing satisfaction level with family visitation improved after implementation of the program based on qualitative responses on the surveys. (A Likert scale was not used on the initial nursing survey, so significance could not be determined.) Our volunteers are also satisfied with their positions; they have all been at their posts for over a year.

Conclusions: Volunteers have been helpful to families by providing necessary support and direction. They have also been helpful to nurses by allowing them to spend more time on patient care and less time controlling flow of visitors. This results in improved satisfaction levels for both families and nurses. This is a cost-effective intervention to assist families of the critically ill. The preliminary success of this program is promising. Volunteers can be used for family assistance in similar settings after careful evaluation of resources.

(May 2006)

CHAPTER 33

The Seed of Research

Cathleen M. Daley

Little did I realize, 28 years ago, that the basic nursing process of assessment, planning, implementation, and evaluation would lead to actual evidence-based nursing research. Seeing a real educational need in my heart failure patients while at their bedsides gave way to ideas.

In 2004, educational handouts were not available for those patients hospitalized with heart failure within my institution. This presented a problem for heart failure patients; could they remember everything I said about their disease process and self-care? The answer was clearly, no! This led me to seek out evidence-based literature, enabling me to coauthor an educational booklet for this cohort. The booklet was concise and easy to read and included a section for daily weight monitoring to encourage patient self-efficacy. Further collaboration with corporate communications led to my obtaining a copyright of this booklet for St. Peter's Hospital. My next question was, How could nursing ensure that the heart failure patient and his family understood the booklet's informational content and that education was given while he was hospitalized? This question was answered when I developed a corresponding interactive discharge sheet. With this done, I still had more questions! What happens to heart failure patients after discharge? What happens when they no longer have home care? How can the heart failure patient and his family be supported in the community? How can I influence these patients at high risk for rehospitalization? My answers to all these questions were as follows: A proposal was given to the cardiac director for the formation of a heart failure support group within the community. Approval was given in March 2005. The first support group meeting was in June 2005 and had 42 attendees, traveling distances of up to 150 miles! The lectures for the attendees were consistent with answering the basic questions such as: What is heart failure? What are the treatment modalities for heart failure? What are the dietary restrictions? What are the exercise essentials? What about smoking cessation? And what are the signs and symptoms that heart failure patients need to report to their healthcare provider?

Soon it was 2006, and again I had more questions! The support group participants were patients with multisystem failure; they had diabetes, atrial fibrillation, renal insufficiency, Chronic Obstructive Pulmonary Disease (COPD), and depression. Their feedback suggested that our lectures go beyond the basics of heart failure education. Yet another question arose within me: Was I truly preventing rehospitalization through education and community support?

Entering 2007, three years after my initial question, there was clear evidence before me that would again formulate a question. Those patients who were consistent in their attendance at the support group had verbalized that they had no rehospitalizations for heart failure. Lifestyle changes were achieved through dietary adherence and medications compliance. Cardiac ejection fractions improved. For example, a 43-year-old female with an ejection fraction initially at 32% in 2005 was at 52% in 2007.

This evidence only led me to ask myself more questions! How could I prove that educating the heart failure patient about his disease process and self-care and supporting him across the continuum from hospital to home were really working?

Where does evidence-based information come from? My answers all led to: *research*! Research would lead me to an evidence-based literature review, testing my hypothesis, and eventually more questions!

So, to answer the question, in August 2007 I developed the heart failure research proposal: "The Effectiveness of In-Hospital Education, Telehealth Homecare and a Heart Failure Support Group: Improve Quality of Life and Decrease the Rate of Hospital Recidivism of the Heart Failure Patient." Full institutional review board approval was obtained on August 8, 2007. This research started on January 1, 2008, and ended on July 1, 2008.

This research will attempt to answer the question of whether we really make a difference when we educate our patients and support them across the continuum. This will, of course, lead back to more questions . . . that will need more answers!

The cycle continues: A simple *need* becomes the *seed* of an *idea* that *grows* to become the tree of *action*. The tree's branches multiply, and the leaves of *evaluation* bloom, fostering *research*!

The Effectiveness of In-Hospital Education: Telehealth Homecare and Heart Failure Support Group: Improve Quality of Life and Decrease the Rate of Hospital Recidivism of the Heart Failure Patient

Cathleen M. Daley, MS, RN

Background:

Financial

Literature indicates that the congestive heart failure (HF) patient in the United States has an exceedingly high readmission rate that reaches 50% by six months, with a projected cost of $7,000 per admission. Approximately 700,000 Medicare recipients are diagnosed annually with congestive heart failure (Miller & Missov, 2001). Heart failure is the most common indication for hospital admission among older adults. Readmissions within three months of hospitalization not only have a negative impact on the HF patient's quality of life but also have a mortality rate of 15% (Blue, et al., 2001).

Rationale

The incidence of heart failure is increasing by 500,000 new cases per year in the United States (Rich, 1997). With each subsequent readmission to the hospital, quality of life for the patient with HF decreases while the mortality rate increases. This project is a response to a documented healthcare problem. Noncompliance with recommended lifestyle changes is estimated to cause 50% of HF rehospitalizations (Caboral & Mitchell, 2003). Education, counseling, and ongoing support for patients with congestive heart failure are necessary for long-term management (Jaarsma, et al., 2004). Intervention during the inpatient phase of HF care provides a significant opportunity to influence a patient's quality of life while preventing a high readmission rate.

Education

Information about diet, smoking cessation, daily weight monitoring, physical activity, medication compliance, and early reporting of worsening signs and symptoms to the patient's healthcare provider can reduce hospital admissions (Anderson, Deepak, Amaoteng-Adjepong, & Zarich, 2005). A demonstration of the relationship between a progressive education program and rate of readmissions will emphasize and identify opportunities to optimize health and decrease overall costs to the healthcare system by disrupting patterns of readmission. This program will offer patients a continuum of care for HF patients. Program education is initiated with the hospitalized HF patient and is followed by telehealth home care at discharge with the additional educational reinforcement through the community-based heart failure support group. The rate of hospital recidivism for this cohort will be compared with each subgroup receiving services of education throughout the continuum.

REFERENCES

Anderson, C., Deepak, B. V., Amaoteng-Adjepong, Y., & Zarich, S. (2005). Benefits of comprehensive inpatient education and discharge planning combined with outpatient support in elderly patients with congestive heart failure. *Congestive Heart Failure, 11*(6), 315–321.

Blue, L., Lang, E., McMurray, J. J. V., Davie, A. P., McDonagh, T. A., Murdoch, R. D., et al. (2001). Randomised controlled trial of specialist nurse intervention in heart failure. *British Medical Journal, 323*(7315), 715–718.

Caboral, M., & Mitchell, J. (2003). New guidelines for heart failure focus on prevention. *The Nurse Practitioner: The American Journal of Primary Health Care, 28*(1), 13, 16, 22–23.

Jaarsma, T., Van Der Wahl, M. H., Hogenhuis, J., Lesman, I., Luttik, M.L., Veeger, M. J., et al. (2004). Design and methodology of the COACH study: A multicenter randomised coordinating study evaluating outcomes of advising and counselling in heart failure. *European Journal of Heart Failure, 6*(2), 227–233.

Miller, L. W., & Missov, E. D. (2001). Epidemiology of heart failure. *Cardiology Clinics, 19*(4), 547–555.

Rich, M. W. (1997). Epidemiology, pathophysiology, and etiology of congestive heart failure in older adults. *Journal of the American Geriatrics Society, 45*(8), 968–974.

CHAPTER 34

Pioneer Nursing Research Team

Steven T. Anderson

Over the last four years, I have had the opportunity and privilege to talk about my professional experience as a primary investigator (PI) for what our institution called a pioneer research team. I thought it would be an easy task to write an essay about a subject that has become less of a career and more of a passion; however, I have struggled to make the topic interesting enough so that others would want to read about it.

Before our team was put together, I had a nursing career that spanned upward of 20 years, six hospitals, one wife, and an untold number of off-shift tours of duty. As a staff nurse, my specialty has always been in emergency nursing, but I have dabbled in management and critical care. It was in the middle of the 1980s when I completed my baccalaureate of science in nursing degree. At the time, I did not understand why I wanted or needed to complete my degree. Unlike many of my colleagues, I have always simply placed "RN" on my name badge. Why? It was more than being too lazy to make the extra effort. I always felt that the alphabet soup after nurses' names was there to impress themselves and other nurses like them. In my mind, a degree never impressed even the most astute of my patients, and I don't remember that it ever made me richer financially, but holding my personal standards higher made me feel richer professionally. My wife always seemed impressed with my nursing degree, but then I think she would have been impressed anyway, which explains our enduring 30-years-plus marriage! In all of my professional years, I have never lost the feeling of awe that I get when a person with diabetes springs to consciousness after a short intravenous drip of dextrose, or when a small child begins play with his toy truck after being dehydrated and recovering with a healthy saline intravenous bolus. The relief expressed on his mother's face—she brought him in just a few hours prior thinking that the worst was happening—is very inspiring. Point being, I now have a similar feeling, having just completed my first research study that has our institution's IRB approval and a plan to publish it in the very near future.

That was the thumbnail version, but like I said, we began this project almost four years ago. Prior to the launching of our team, our hospital had already been working to establish guidelines for pioneer nursing research teams. All of this was part of an institutional goal to become a designated Magnet hospital. Possibly because of the nature of our department's operations, the enthusiastic support of our department's leadership, or a combination of both, our emergency department and three other nursing units were selected to be the pioneer research teams. I was late to come aboard and only became actively involved after another member left the team. I was asked to participate, I think, mostly because my schedule allowed me to be at every meeting (which by itself was an asset), and later on I became the PI for the same reason. I have to say that I was reluctant at first. I saw research as endless literature reviews of other people's research but never getting an opportunity to actually identify a problem, ask a question about it, and then develop a study to find the answer. When it became clear that we would be able to develop our own *little piece of science* for the whole body of nursing, it started to get exciting.

The process was simple:

1. Only staff nurses chose the questions and developed the studies to answer them. Our leadership offered suggestions and guidance to aid us through bureaucratic hurdles and logistical support.
2. Meetings would be held every month for one hour, and all work would be completed during the meeting, which meant that there would be no off-time obligation to the project.
3. Each pioneer research team would have a voting representative on the hospital research council and would keep the council updated.

The enthusiasm started to change the rules slightly. Team members eventually decided to meet more often than monthly. Literature reviews became too labor intensive to accomplish in the hour designated for the meetings and were preventing the completion of other work. The team decided to perform literature searches on off-duty time. This same attitude proved very helpful when it came time to collect data, because it eventually became clear that data collection could not be done by a staff nurse on duty. We had established a work ethic early in the process; the completion of this study would have been jeopardized had such a work ethic not been in place.

Weeks and months elapsed as we worked out what would be studied and the IRB protocol, and assured that everything was in place to begin our data collection. Though somewhat expected, our Magnet visit was looming. The exact date had not yet been set, but we all knew that it would be sooner rather than later. In an exercise to prepare for the Magnet visit, a consultant was hired to preevaluate our chances of success. To make this brief, let us say that our research program lacked what was necessary to be designated a Magnet hospital. As we sat in our boardroom, we heard from the consultant that all of our good work was probably not enough—not because the work was not stellar, but because it had not been done long enough and because most of our pioneer teams had not yet received IRB approval. The meeting ended not with long-faced dejected researchers, but just the opposite. I, like many of my counterparts, quickly began to pull out all the stops. We were literally making plans right outside the boardroom door to make this project a success. We could not do anything about the past, but we were determined to make sure that we did not fail because we had not done everything in our power to get our data collected and studies IRB approved. Enough drama—our hospital was Magnet designated, and our research program was highlighted in the designation as one of the reasons that our hospital received the award!

Where are we now? All of our research pioneer teams have completed their studies or are nearing completion. One has already published a research article in a national nursing publication, and our team is ready to publish. Four new research teams from different nursing units are beginning the research process. Our team set the bar high, and we encourage our successors to keep the standards high. As staff nurses we have had the opportunity to interact with colleagues in our institution through public speaking at monthly Nursing Grand Rounds and poster presentations. We have traveled across our state, speaking at nursing leadership conferences and making poster presentations at our state-supported university, and we have participated in and presented at national research conferences. Our schedule for the coming year indicates that we will be well traveled and will continue to garner respect and prestige for our research, which is undoubtedly on the leading edge of nursing research outside of an academic institution.

As a PI, I personally have gained a whole new perspective on the workings of my hospital. Some examples:

1. Before this all began, I liked to joke that I could not even spell IRB, but I have had to present changes in our research protocol to the IRB and argue for the approval of the changes to our protocol.
2. A new document was needed so that our researchers could administer a study agent—essentially a doctor's order. This new document needed approval by a special committee before it could become an official part of the medical record. I had no idea that there was a special committee that had to approve new documents. After submitting our newly proposed document and getting its approval, I am now on good terms with that committee.
3. The research council needed an icon for all forms, correspondence, posters, and so on for research activities. I suddenly found out that I needed to be a graphic artist. The design I created, a simple apple with the initials *NR* inside the core, is on everything that leaves our hospital

for other research conferences, along with a catch phrase: *Nursing Research Is the Core of Evidence-Based Nursing Practice.* It has received good reviews, and other professionals have asked for our permission to use it.

4. I will take the reins as committee chairman of the hospital research council next year. *Networking* is more of an action word to me than a concept these days. I am hoping for a very productive year as chairman, and I am already building a coalition to assure that success.

I mentioned earlier the awe I experienced from the recovery of a person with diabetes who suffered from hypoglycemia and the child who was dehydrated. I still feel pride in being a part of all that, but this research study has to be my greatest work. It is my legacy, but I have another one in me. I will start over again in the spring!

Acknowledgment: I would like to express my warmest regards and gratitude to my research team: Jean Cockrell, BSN, RN; Elizabeth Murphy, BSN, RN; and Patricia Beller, PhD, RN. I also would like to extend a special expression of gratitude to Joan Cederna-Moss, MSN, RN, for mentoring us through the nursing research process. Thank you to our then-director Pat Nelson, MSN, RN, and our then-clinical manager, Liz Domanski, BSN, RN, whose support made our research team possible. Let me thank our new director, Mary Lynn Smith, MSN, RN, for her continued support of our program and for giving us almost carte blanche authority to do whatever was necessary. Finally, I want to thank our chief nursing officer, Mary Lou Powell, for her vision and insightful goal of seeing us through to Magnet designation. Through the many days and months, we went through more than we ever expected. I hold each of you in the highest esteem, and I am humbled by your professionalism.

Administration of Local Anesthetic Agents to Decrease Pain Associated with Peripheral Vascular Access

Steven T. Anderson, BSN, RN

Purpose: This study compares a variety of local anesthetic agents and the administration methods prior to starting an intravenous device to determine which method is most comfortable for the patient.

Design: A randomized double-blind placebo pretest–posttest experimental design was used to compare five treatment groups.

Setting: This study was conducted in an emergency department of a 388-bed community-based hospital in the southeastern region of the United States, with an average of 52,000 visits per year.

Sample: This study used a convenience sample of patients admitted to the emergency department who required insertion of an IV device. Inclusion criteria were: age > 18 years; vein characteristics that would accommodate a 20-G or larger gauge IV device; hemodynamic stability; oriented to self and environment; and an antecubital fossa, hand, or forearm IV catheter site. Exclusion criteria were allergy to any components of the anesthetic agents; history of poor venous access or IV drug abuse; venipuncture procedure within 24 hours; potential psychiatric disturbance; pregnancy; and/or history of peripheral neuropathies. Sample size was based on power analysis for F tests for a five-group design, an effect size of 0.35, power of 0.80, and alpha = 0.05. The five treatment groups were composed of a total 86 study subjects (anesthetic spray; placebo spray; anesthetic intradermal injection; placebo intradermal injection; and a control group with no local anesthetic agent). Approval was obtained from the institution's investigational review board prior to data collection.

Methodology: Dependent variables were the patient's pain level at the IV insertion site before, and one minute after, local anesthetic agent application, and three minutes after IV catheter insertion and the nurse's rating of vein quality. Confounding variables were catheter size, successful cannulation of the vein, and difficulty of IV insertion. Randomization into treatment groups was done with a computer-generated random number table. The primary dependent variable was the patient's pain level at the IV insertion site before and after local anesthetic agent application, and after IV catheter insertion.

Results: Anesthetic intradermal injection was found to have significantly higher pain ratings one minute after application as compared with the other treatment groups ($F_{4,79} = 3.76$, $p = 0.008$). Pain ratings three minutes after IV insertion were found to be similar for the five treatment groups ($F_{4,71} = 0.79$, $p = 0.533$). Significant decreases in vein quality after intradermal injections for both anesthetic and placebo groups were found as compared with the topical sprays and control groups (chi-square = 16.4, $df = 8$, $p = 0.037$).

Conclusions: The use of an intradermal anesthetic agent prior to IV insertion caused a significant increase in pain immediately after administration, and degradation of vein quality. Pain scores after IV insertion were not significantly different for the five groups.

CHAPTER 35

Me Do Research? Are You Kidding?

Lou Ann Jones

When I was an undergraduate nursing student in the early 1980s, my professor's lectures on research were centered on, "What is the question?" I can remember thinking to myself, *I don't know the question or the answer, is that not what I am here to learn?* After working at the bedside for many years, I can finally say that I understand what they were trying to teach me. Working as a staff nurse and spending hours with patients force you to evaluate constantly why you do things a certain way and to consider alternative ways to current practice. So, when I was approached by another master's-prepared nurse with a similar question about practice, I started to seriously consider the question, *Could I be the one to conduct nursing research and provide the answers?*

My nursing colleague was a member of the nursing research council at the time and invited me to the monthly meeting as a guest. That was over four years ago, and with the help and encouragement of the director of nursing research at the hospital where I work, I am still hooked on nursing research. Every nurse is taught from early in his or her career to think about the "whys" of events. Doing nursing research is taking that critical thinking skill and formalizing it into a process that can be measured and evaluated using mathematical equations.

Doing nursing research was very rewarding once I figured out how to answer the question, "What is the question?" Of course, it takes lots of support from colleagues, friends, and family to get you through the rough spots, but in the end, improving patient care and making nurses more successful in what they do is what it is all about. I also had the opportunity to present the results of this study at national conferences, including the National Institutes of Health.

Acknowledgment: I would like to extend my warmest thanks to colleagues who have supported me on my research journey, especially the members of the staff of the Inova Heart and Vascular Institutes, Loudoun Campus. Dr. Gabel Speroni's encouragement and sense of humor helped keep me focused on reaching my goal even when I thought I would not achieve it.

A Prospective Randomized Study Evaluating the Flushing Procedure Using 0.9% Sodium Chloride versus Heparin Lock Flush in Peripherally Inserted Central Catheters Combined with a Fluid Displacement Luer-Activated Device

Linda Bowers, MSN, APRN, BC, OCN; Karen Gabel Speroni, PhD, RN; Lou Ann Jones, MSN, APRN, BC; and Martin Atherton, DrPH

Purpose: This study was conducted with the objective of obtaining evidence-based practice data that compared the occlusion rates of two flushing solutions, normal saline (NS) and heparinized saline (HS), when used to flush peripherally inserted central catheters (PICCs) with luer-activated devices.

Design: In this prospective randomized study of 102 subjects with single-lumen peripherally inserted central catheters with positive pressure luer-activated devices, two flushing solution groups were compared for their effect on occlusion rates.

Methods: Patients who met eligibility criteria were enrolled in the study over a 2-year period between 2004 and 2006. Subjects were randomized in a 1:1 ratio to one of the following flushing solution groups:

- NS (0.9% sodium chloride injections, USP, Abbott Laboratories, North Chicago, IL)
- HS (heparin lock flush USP, 100 USP Units/mL heparin sodium, 5 mL in a 6-mL vial), American Pharmaceutical Partners, East Schaumburg, IL)

Study-related data were recorded at four time points: insertion, flushing, study termination, and occlusion if it occurred.

Results: Sixty percent were female in the NS group, and 40% were female in the HS group (X-square = 3.9, $p < 0.05$). For both groups, the average age was 54 years, and the majority were Whites with admitting diagnoses of infection: muscular/skeletal, respiratory, genito-urinary/renal, or gastrointestinal.

There was a total of three PICC line occlusions, all of which occurred in the NS group (NS = 6%; HS = 0%). Nurses performed a total of 437 flushing procedures in the NS group and 354 in the HS group. The average number of flushes per subject was 8.6 in the NS group versus 6.9 in the HS group. The average number of flushes per day in the NS group was 4.1 versus 2.3 in the HS group (t test = 24.6, $p < 0.0001$).

The average duration of the PICC line was 2.1 (range 0.25–25.5) days for the NS group and 2.9 (0.25–40.0) days for the HS group (t test = 0.8, $p = 0.2$). The primary reason for flushing was to provide medication (75% in the NS group and 65% in the HS group), followed by daily flushing and blood draws.

All three occlusions occurred among elderly (average age = 66 years) White females admitted for infection or respiratory disorders. The average duration of the catheter was 10.3 days. Patency was restored for two of the three occlusions using alteplase.

Conclusions: From an evidence-based practice perspective, the results did not support a change to the hospital's standard nursing procedure to eliminate the use of HS. However, the differences in flushing solution occlusion rates are economically significant, because occlusions can result in the requirement for PICC line replacement. The replacement charge for a PICC line in interventional radiology is more than US $1,900 in the hospital where the research was conducted.

REFERENCES

Bowers, L., Speroni, K. G., Jones, L. A., & Atherton, M. (2008). Comparison of occlusion rates by flushing solutions for peripherally inserted central catheters with positive pressure luer-activated devices. *Journal of Infusion Nursing, 31*(1) 22–27.

CHAPTER 36

My Experience in Nursing Research

Diane Braun

Although I had experience in clinical research prior to joining the nursing research council at my institution, I had very little experience in nursing research. I developed a strong belief in the impact that nursing care has on patient outcomes because of my many years working as a medical-surgical nurse, and then as a clinical research coordinator. The physiologic and the psychological healing that take place every day in health care are tremendously dependent on good nursing care. Nurses do a lot for patients and their families, which has traditionally been based on our training, intuition, and instinct.

For example, during the nine years that I worked as a nurse in an intensive care unit/critical care unit, I compulsively did my best to keep patients clean. Providing oral care to my patients was a priority for me, especially for my patients who were intubated. I am grateful now that research has proved that fastidious oral hygiene is important in preventing ventilator-associated pneumonias. Now, as nurses, we have objective data to support what I always "felt" was correct, even though there was no set standard or policy to support this. On the other hand, I have learned that bathing patients too often with soap can be harmful to their skin. The pH can be shifted too high from the normally acidic pH, which may affect the normal bacterial flora of the skin. I realize that my instinct was overzealous in regard to bathing, now that there is objective information to prove this. The point I am making is that nursing as a profession needs objective data and organized studies to guide our best practices and help us prioritize our care and time management. Suffice it to say that I am a strong proponent of research and evidence-based practice.

My recent experience with nursing research was prompted by a requirement for my master's program to design and, if possible, implement an improvement-oriented innovation at my institution. I consulted my director and was encouraged to join the nursing research council of Advocate Christ Medical Center and Hope Children's Hospital in the summer of 2005. Our medical center had just recently been awarded Magnet status, and the nursing research council had recently formed to develop and facilitate nursing research. I was quickly welcomed onto the committee and invited to be the lead principal investigator in a project that was in the planning stages to promote nursing research.

A nurse researcher consultant from a local university who had previously assisted our institution with our Magnet application and approval process suggested a previously reported model project for the group to use in planning the project.

Using the Great American Cookie Experiment as a model, our nursing research council decided to conduct a similar, but not identical, project. The objective was to engage staff nurses throughout our hospital in a fun and educational introduction to research. After much debate and consideration, we made the decision to conduct a hand lotion sampling project. A subcommittee convened that, among other details, ironed out and named the project "Softening the Essentials of Nursing Research: The Great Lotion Promotion."

A follow-up survey to the Great Lotion Promotion was conducted in 2006 to evaluate the effectiveness of the initial housewide clinical staff nurse educational endeavor. There was a good response rate, with approximately 20% of the surveys returned. The postsurvey results showed a positive trend regarding interest, knowledge, and comfort levels with nursing research in the comparison of nurses who participated in the Lotion Promotion with nurses who did not participate.

My experience of being involved with a process demonstration project at my institution showed me the tremendous time commitment that is involved in nursing research. The original Lotion Promotion project, which included almost 20 members of the council, had an energizing and binding impact on the group. When I conducted the follow-up survey by myself (to have a conclusion for my capstone project), I longed for the assistance of the group.

My conclusion here is that there is strength in numbers. I recommend engaging a committee; I found using a committee to be a much more enjoyable and efficient method to conduct a project. My other advice is to pick a project that is relevant to your institution because that will provide the motivation and excitement to complete the project and discover the results. Regardless of the time, effort, and costs involved in organizing and conducting nursing research, I believe that the beneficial empowerment to our profession is priceless.

Acknowledgment: I'd like to extend my warmest thanks to colleagues on the nursing research council of Advocate Christ Medical Center and Hope Children's Hospital who have supported me on my research journey. In particular, I'd like to voice my appreciation for their support to Dr. Wendy Micke; Dr. Denise Angst; Donna Ellis, MSN, RN, APN; Beth Fournier, BSN; and Dr. Cheryl LeFavier. Without their encouragement and assistance, this project never would have been completed.

Softening the Essentials of Nursing Research: The Great Lotion Promotion

Diane Braun, BSN, MA, CCRP; Donna Ellis, MSN, RN, APN;
Beth Fournier, BSN; Wendy Tuzik-Micek, DNSc, RN;
Denise Angst, DNSc, RN; Ted Temkin, PhD; and Cheryl Lefaiver, PhD, RN

Advanced practice and staff nurses may perceive many barriers to conducting research and incorporating it into their practice. The nursing research council at a Midwestern Medical Center implemented a fun demonstration study designed to engage and educate nurses about the fundamentals of a nursing research project. Using the Great American Cookie Experiment as a model, a housewide double-blind randomized study was conducted to assess nursing perceptions of hand lotion.

Researchers approached nurses on individual nursing units at varying days and times over a 4-week period. Nurse participants signed an informed consent, completed a demographic survey, and selected a randomization card to first receive Lotion A on either the right hand or left hand; Lotion B was then applied to the other hand. During the lotion application, researchers described the steps of the nursing research process using a preprinted research process flow chart. Finally, participants completed a survey about their lotion preference, which included questions about the moisture, residue, and scent, on a 4-point scale from *poor* to *very good*. Participants also answered one question about the overall preference of the lotions. Descriptive statistics were used for the demographic data, and chi-square and Wilcoxon signed-rank analysis were used for the comparison of the two lotions.

A total of 500 nurses participated, representing 25% of the hospital's employed nurses. The majority were female (87%), were aged 41–50 years, and had less than ten years of experience. Overall, nurses reported a significant ($p < 0.01$) preference for Lotion B. Comparisons for lotion characteristics showed that a significant ($p < 0.01$) difference existed for lotion scent only. No significant difference was found for lotion moisture or residue. Unblinding revealed Lotion A as the lotion currently supplied to the medical center. Because

Lotion B was preferred, a recommendation will be made to nursing administration to adjust the lotion supplied on the units.

In conclusion, the researchers achieved the objective of reaching a large portion of the current nursing staff and exposing them to the research process. Nurses were receptive to the information, enjoyed the simple experiment, and appreciated that they were contacted on the unit level.

CHAPTER 37

The Defining Moment That Led Me into Research

Suzanne S. Clark

Prior to doing my research study, "Trends and Factors in Blood Pressure in Hyperbaric Medicine," I had been asked numerous times by patients undergoing hyperbaric oxygen treatments about why there was an increase in their blood pressures after their treatments. I provided patient teaching regarding increased blood pressure and vasoconstriction, but I could not explain why it does not always occur during every treatment. I had heard about evidence-based practice research being done at our hospital, so in 2005 I approached my manager about possibly doing a study. At that time, I had also attended performance improvement training classes at the hospital, which helped me to define what factors and trends to look at when observing changes in blood pressure. My manager felt that it was a good idea for a study and approached the nurse researcher at our hospital. I had also spoken to the hyperbaric unit practicing physicians, who felt that the study would be a valid one.

At that point, I felt both excited and overwhelmed at the possibilities. I was not sure how receptive the patients would be about participating in the study. The additional time to wait and have their blood pressure taken again after the treatment, as well as taking an anxiety questionnaire prior to the treatment, may be viewed negatively. Was the staff member going to follow through with the required data collection to do the study? Would there be a large enough sample?

Just prior to starting the research, there was a safety inspection for accreditation by the Undersea and Hyperbaric Medicine Society. During the inspection, it was discussed that I would be conducting the study, and they asked me questions about how it would be done. At that time, I felt intimidated as I spoke to the inspectors. I remember feeling unsure of myself and unsure of how they were going to react. I felt more confident as I spoke to them and saw how receptive they were.

After data collection on the first ten patients was completed and analyzed, an abstract was submitted to the Undersea Hyperbaric Medicine Society for the scientific meeting in Maui. It took approximately two months to hear whether it would be accepted. The nurse researcher, the nurse manager, and I were hoping for a poster presentation. To our surprise, the abstract was accepted for both a poster and an oral presentation. Then I really became nervous. I knew I could do it if I set my mind to it, but I had never done one before. I was really concerned about whether the professionals at the meeting would be interested in my topic or in hearing me speak. I practiced at home in front of the mirror over and over again. Then I repeatedly practiced in front of the computer using the PowerPoint presentation. The presentation was successful.

The advice I would give anyone interested in doing evidence-based research is to pick a topic that you feel could affect how you practice nursing. Ask others for their input and whether they feel the study has validity. Also, talk to others about their studies and how they came up with their ideas. At my hospital, Morristown Memorial Hospital, there are short meetings during lunch, called "lunch and learn." These meetings allow nurses who do research to present their studies and receive feedback from their colleagues. Before going to Maui for the Undersea Hyperbaric Medicine Society scientific meeting, I gave my oral presentation. Doing that presentation increased my confidence level and further improved my presentation skills as more experienced colleagues responded with even more suggestions.

Currently, I am completing the blood pressure study with a total of 30 subjects to see if the results are the same as with the first ten. As for pursuing evidence-based research, the defining moment for me was the patient asking me why.

Acknowledgment: I would like to acknowledge and thank Dr. Susan Fowler, nurse researcher, and Denise Fochesto, nurse manager, for giving me guidance and support as a novice researcher. Without their interest, the study would not have been a success.

Trends and Factors in Blood Pressure in Hyperbaric Oxygen Treatment

Suzanne S. Clark, RN, ACHRN; and Susan Fowler, PhD, MMH

Introduction: Clinically it is noted that blood pressure (BP) is often elevated after hyperbaric oxygen (HBO) treatment in patients with and without a history of hypertension. Even though blood pressure increases and heart rate decreases, the cardiac output stays the same. National standards are lacking for BP monitoring and management in patients undergoing HBO therapy. Standards generally acknowledge that a clinical history should be obtained before treatment, and during therapy, physiologic and clinical monitoring is done and side and adverse effects monitored with reassessment of the patient as indicated. The purpose of this study is to investigate trends in BP following HBO treatments and to explore factors that may influence BP in patients undergoing HBO.

Materials and Methods: This is a descriptive correlation study involving a convenience sample of adults ($N = 10$), inpatients and outpatients. Subjects will complete the state portion of the State-Trait Anxiety Inventory (STAI) (Y Form) before the second through sixth treatment (five occasions). Subjects will undergo HBO treatment as prescribed, and vital signs will be taken according to routine established in the HBO area, but the patient will be lying down. If systolic blood pressure (SBP) is > 20 mmHg above baseline and/or diastolic blood pressure (DBP) is > 10 mmHg above baseline, the patient will be asked questions regarding possible symptoms and pain and be instructed to lie quietly for five minutes; BP will be repeated.

Results: Six patients had episodes of elevated SBP after treatment. In two of these six, SBP was elevated more than 50% of the time (three to five treatments), and neither had a history of Hypertension (HTN). The other four patients had a history of HTN and were taking medications before treatment. Four patients did not experience elevated SBPs. Eight patients experienced episodes of elevated DBP posttreatment. In one of these eight, DBP was elevated more than 50% of the time (three to five treatments). This individual did not have a history of HTN and experienced a similar increase in SBPs. In the other seven patients, four had a history of HTN and were taking medications. Only two patients did not experience elevated DBPs. Half of the patients (five) experienced both elevations in SBP and DBP. Individual anxiety scores ranged from 20 to 49 (possible 20–80). Mean scores over time ranged from 20 to 48, with females exhibiting higher anxiety scores (21–48). No male indicated a score above 28. Fifty percent ($N = 5$) had anxiety scores from 20 to 28. There was no identified trend in anxiety scores from session to session. In four of the ten patients (40%), the anxiety score was lower at the final session (Session 5) compared with the first session. Only one patient identified pain during the procedure, and during this one episode, his anxiety score was highest; although both his SBP and DBP increased, they were not above the acceptable range.

Conclusions: One-third of the time, posttreatment BP was elevated above pretreatment levels, but patients did not experience S&S related to this elevation. Most of the time (65%), BP decreased after five minutes of rest. Half of the patients experienced BP elevations. One-half to two-thirds of the time, these elevations occurred in patients with a history of HTN. Elevations in DBP were more frequent in patients without a history of HTN. Few patients experienced pain during treatments. Females were more anxious than males with no identified trend over time. Highest anxiety occurred in a female without a history of HTN; she had claustrophobia and had taken sedatives prior to HBO treatment. Both SBPs (nine times) and DBPs (seven times) were elevated more often in patients with higher mean anxiety levels. DBP increased more often (six times) in patients with low anxiety as compared with SBP (two times). Nurses need to continue to assess BP before and after HBO treatments; assess anxiety and offer psychosocial support; and recommend five minutes of rest after posttreatment BP elevations.

CHAPTER 38

The Ice Study: Quenching the Thirst

Nancy B. Hutchison and Megan E. Brunson

Overcome with patients' discomfort related to thirst post open-heart surgery, several nurses created this research project as a result of discussing the differences between patient care in dealing with the "thirsty, dry-mouthed" patients. The need to evaluate this issue was multifactorial. It is a huge issue for patient comfort and can turn into a battle of wills involving the nurse at the bedside, the patient, and the family in order to balance the patient's safety with oral comfort. Patient safety was a big concern in terms of avoiding vomiting to prevent graft dehiscence by increased intrathoracic pressure. The surgeons were willing to try to study this issue after obtaining consent from the whole group of physicians.

The project started with eight to ten RNs, and not much thought was given to who would do what. We were excited and eager to begin preliminary data gathering and review any published data. We felt very little pressure, because each of us would be part of the greater whole, and the clinical nurse specialist (CNS) of the unit would put everything together. At this time, we were part of the team interested in this study but not the primary investigators.

The CNS/primary investigator resigned from the hospital. The loss of this individual created a large hole in the continuation of the research because many of the RNs on this project worked weekends and nights. The loss of a full-time daily person with flexible hours was very dramatic. It stalled the research, and the rest of the team was unmotivated to continue. However, the two of us decided to continue, and we revised the final proposal during our personal time. We formally submitted it to the nursing research council during one of their quarterly meetings.

At this time, Nancy was asked to assume the role of primary investigator. However, the work was so overwhelming that it required the hands of two people. We were approved by the Center for Nursing Excellence for budgeted resource hours to be paid, and secretarial services would be provided. We applied for a small in-hospital grant. With these things in mind, we talked to the research team. It appeared that the study could go forward as planned. We soon became highly burdened with the institutional review board (IRB) paperwork and the details involved in HIPAA regulations even though we would not be passing out medications or doing procedures on patients. The IRB process took four months.

The next step was to order graduated cups to fill with ice for the patients. We were overcome with red tape when the hospital attempted to encourage us to use their vendor. However, we explained that we could obtain the cups at a less expensive rate through another supplier. Megan had to place the cups on her credit card and then hope to be paid back at a later date. We also were forced to purchase Sprite for the patients, although initially we were told that we could order it through patient nutritional services without difficulty.

Our biggest challenge was obtaining informed consent from the patients preoperatively. Because stable patients (who were good candidates) are admitted early on the day of surgery, we had a difficult time recruiting subjects. The in-house patients were generally unstable, which meant that they were unlikely to meet study criteria post-op. The changes in the study team personnel made this extremely difficult, because we had no RN working routine day hours who could leave her assignment in a busy intensive care unit (ICU) to go and consent patients for the next day. As a result, it took nearly six months to recruit ten patients per group, for a total of 40. Our unit does a high volume of at least 25 heart surgeries a week; we should have been able to obtain these patients in less than a month. We also were not reimbursed for any research time or secretarial assistance even though we were approved for these costs prior to the study.

Research is a slow process, and it was difficult to change our thinking, considering that we work in a fast-paced ICU with an "instant fix" mentality. We had to think outside the box and learn the system over time. We were up for the challenge, because we wanted to make a name for our unit. To continue this study with a larger sample, we would have to clarify financial and secretarial support consistently.

The project ended with two RNs (from the original group of ten nurses) who were determined to find the answers. Research takes persistence and determination, because one is guaranteed to have obstacles that one can only imagine. However, the ability to safely meet the needs of our patients' requests for fluid versus ice chips was achieved.

Acknowledgment: We would like to acknowledge our deepest appreciation to the following members of our bedside research team in the cardiovascular ICU of St. Joseph's of Atlanta: Ann Marie Madden, Tina Taylor, Joyce Crook, Rebecca Reece, Fang Jiang, and Cheryl Bittel. We would also like to thank Diana Meeks-Sgonstrom and Susan Beard for their time and guidance.

To Determine Which of Four Interventions Postoperative Cardiac Surgery Patients Perceive as Best Quenching Their Thirst with the Least Amount of Nausea and Vomiting

Nancy B. Hutchison, MS, RN, CCRN; and
Megan E. Brunson, BSN, RN, CCRN-CSC

Purpose: To determine the best practice of four interventions attempted with post-op cardiac surgery patients that would best quench their thirst and simultaneously reduce nausea and vomiting.

Need for Study: We have had much internal debate over the substance, as well as timing and amount, to initially provide patients with oral hydration postextubation from cardiac surgery. To date, no study has evaluated the amount or type of oral hydration initiated in postoperative cardiac patients. Nurses who fear nausea and vomiting tend to give approximately 30 cc of ice chips, and nothing more, for the first 12 hours postextubation. Other nurses provide patients with ample amounts of fluids, to include ice chips and water as tolerated. Both interventions have mixed results that have not been formally evaluated. Evidence-based practice is required to provide interventions that will meet the need for patient satisfaction while ensuring the highest standard of care. The complaints from patients include thirst, extremely dry mouth, and postextubation oral condition, otherwise known as morning breath.

Design: The method for this research study was a randomized comparison of four separate groups. Patients were consented prior to surgery, and interventions took place in the first 12 hours postextubation. The group assignment was determined by a random pull out of a box as the patient was admitted to the cardiovascular intensive care unit (CVICU).

Sample: The pilot study involved a random sample of 40 patients (four groups of ten).

Setting: The study took place in a 410-bed acute care hospital that performs more than 1,500 cardiac procedures annually. An average range of postoperative admissions is from two to 14 patients per day. The CVICU recovery areas are two large six-bed open rooms where the patients will stay less than 24 hours before transferring to the cardiac telemetry unit.

Groups:

1. Group 1 received 30 cc/hr, or less, of ice chips.
2. Group 2 received ice chips as desired up to 120 cc/hr.
3. Group 3 received water at room temperature, as desired, up to 120 cc/hr.
4. Group 4 received up to 120 cc/hr of Diet Sprite.

Data Collection: The data collection tool collected information on patients' blood pressure, their medications, and pain. Previous studies have indicated that postoperative nausea and vomiting can be caused by postoperative pain, anticholinergenics, and hypotension. The data collection tool was developed by the research team after the review of the literature and input from experts in the field. It was then given to expert nurses to review to ensure it was clear to the subjects.

Results: Data analysis showed no statistically significant difference in the vomiting rates of all four groups. The patient satisfaction scores were higher in the patients who received 120 cc/hr of any fluid as compared with ice chips only.

Ethical Considerations: Approval of the nursing research council at Saint Joseph's Hospital of Atlanta and the IRB was obtained.

(2006–2007)

CHAPTER 39

Awakened to Research
by Howard's Awakening

Sharon Truitt

I have worked at the bedside as a critical care nurse for 20 years. During much of that time, my only involvement with nursing research had been the presentation of case studies to my nursing colleagues on our unit. During these patient care conferences, I would present the details of a patient's diagnosis and treatment. These conferences were an opportunity for me to share my experience regarding a particularly challenging and complex patient situation with nurses on the unit. Through these experiences, I learned how to research information and gather pertinent data from the patient's chart and other sources. Even though I felt positive about providing the safest and best care to my patients, I did not envision participating in research beyond these efforts.

That all changed when I met Howard. Howard was a 71-year-old male who was noted to have EKG changes during preadmission testing for eye surgery. A heart catherization revealed triple vessel disease. He had a medical history of diabetes with neuropathy, hypertension, and a positive family cardiac history. Because he was asymptomatic, he had a difficult decision to make regarding whether he should have cardiac surgery. He opted to proceed with coronary artery bypass graft surgery.

From the beginning of his postoperative course, his recovery was far from normal. Open heart surgery may be routine these days, but as Howard's case illustrates, each individual's course of recovery can be very different. On the day of his surgery, per hospital protocol, his endotracheal tube was removed. After its removal, Howard became lethargic. An arterial blood gas showed respiratory acidosis, and reversal agents were not effective; Howard needed to be reintubated. He showed gradual improvement over the next three days. However, I noticed that he became somnolent for hours after a dose of Zofran, which caused concern both for his family and for me. However, he was subsequently transferred to the post-op floor in stable condition.

On post-op Day 7, Howard received a dose of Ambien. Within 15 minutes, he became apneic, bradycardic, and unresponsive. He returned to the cardiothoracic intensive care unit (CTICU) after being resuscitated. Howard was fully vented and unresponsive, even to painful stimuli. He was sent for a stat CT scan of his head. The scan showed no abnormality, but his EEG showed slowing consistent with encephalopathy.

During the time he spent in the cardiac ICU, Howard had alternating periods of unresponsiveness as he received Haldol for restlessness and agitation. Howard did manage to get off the vent again. He was on Dopamine for management of blood pressure and a Lasix drip for fluid overload. Antibiotics were initiated for a lower lobe infiltrate, and he needed aggressive nasotracheal suctioning. Multisystem organ failure was diagnosed due to elevated liver function tests, and creatinine of 3.1 requiring dialysis and pneumonia. What went wrong?

The neurologist diagnosed anoxic encephalopathy. However, I knew that he was awake after his "downtime" from the resuscitation. The physicians attributed his mental status condition to a metabolic disorder. I felt strongly that we were missing something; it was clear to me that not all the puzzle pieces were fitting together. I recalled this patient's journey from the operating room, returning from the code blue and lying in the CTICU in multisystem failure. I was convinced that his reaction to medications was not normal. I encouraged the doctors to discontinue anything that might be making him sleepy. I then decided to research this patient's medications. With further investigation, I found that Howard was receiving Trileptal, Haldol, Reglan, and Zofran. All these medications can contribute to lethargy, dysarthria, and sedation. Could Howard be suffering from the compound side effects of these medications?

Through collaboration with the intensivist and pharmacist, we researched the metabolism and interaction of different drugs, as well as the liver enzymes and factors that interfere with excretion of drugs. With this evidence, these medications were discontinued. Howard began to have periods of consciousness and audible speech. Throughout this time, his wife and children were stressed over the long stay and the multiple complications that their loved one was suffering. As we continued to provide comprehensive nursing care, Howard made a remarkable recovery. I will never forget the day I walked Howard around the unit for the first time. As we were walking around the hallway, his wife came in and panicked because he wasn't in the room. To her delight, he was ambulating into the room behind her.

This was the catalyst for my desire to learn more and educate others. I prepared the information for a presentation at Medical Education Day in 2003. Prior to this year, only physicians, clinical nurse specialists, and educators would have done this collection of data and presented them. I used supporting data from recent articles as I gave this case study. When I had Howard stand in the back of the room at the end of my speech, the whole room cheered. I received an award for the Best Allied Health presentation.

The importance of this scenario was that I became more involved with and inquisitive about each patient and procedure. Coworkers would recall my presentation and comment that their patient seemed to be having symptoms similar to the patient I talked about. Physicians respected me and listened to potential improvements to care.

I believe strongly in continuing education by maintaining my certification as a critical care registered nurse (CCRN), but as Howard's story illustrates, researching and using evidence at the bedside has a profound impact on patient care and is a nursing intervention that can make a real difference in the lives of our patients. Just as Howard woke up from his drug-induced encephalopathy, I woke up and saw the possibilities that nursing research has for me as a staff nurse. I realized that I had embraced a very limited view of what nurses can do at the bedside for their patients. Nursing research opened up a whole new way of thinking about patient care.

As a result of this experience, I became the inaugural chairperson of the nurse practice council, which led to joining the research roundtable. Not being a bachelor's-prepared nurse, I did not think research was feasible. The roundtable is a collaboration of senior nursing students at Messiah College and staff nurses at Pinnacle Health to find best practices. Managers, staff development instructors, and clinical nurse specialists facilitate the research as the group develops a question and focuses on an area of interest. After reviewing the literature, these groups have made changes in policy based on the evidence. Being part of the research roundtable and the research council makes my practice more meaningful. Decisions are made not only by those in administrative positions, but also by those performing the tasks at the bedside.

All nurses have concerns about providing appropriate care and questions about the best ways to do procedures. It is exciting to know that our facility offers several avenues to find the answers. Whether research roundtable, research council, or research fellowship, we the bedside nurses have the potential to positively impact our patient outcomes. If you think things can be done a better way, do not hesitate to get involved in finding the answers. My professional development has benefited, and patient care has improved because of my research experience.

Acknowledgment: Many thanks to Trish Benner, MSN, CNS, who gave me the help and encouragement to present my findings and get involved in the research roundtable, and to Liz Burdick, BSN, nurse manager, for her never-ending support. I am also grateful for the energy I have received from Rhonda Maneval, EdD, RN who is the most spirited, passionate researcher I have found.

CHAPTER 40

Nursing Research—"Just Do It"

Brigitte Taylor

Research has always been an item on my list of things to do in my nursing career. I would read research articles and want to understand how a research project was actually started, assembled, and completed. I was in awe of those who were able to participate in research studies. I wanted to have the opportunity to be involved in the process at least once in my career.

The initial process includes gathering ideas for a research project, writing the protocol, and submitting it to the institutional review board for approval. Then, you are finally able to consent and collect data. This has proved to be an eye-opening experience.

At the Birthing Inn, we were curious about the breastfeeding experience for patients after their discharge. We wanted to answer these questions: How long did patients breastfeed? Did they fulfill their breastfeeding expectations? If their expectations were not met, were there any outside factors that may have contributed to their breastfeeding goals not being fulfilled? These factors could include little family support and work-related factors.

We are still in the process of data collection. So far, I have found research to be very labor intensive. While getting caught up with how things are completed, you essentially become obsessed with everything related to the project. It is truly a satisfying experience when you can start a research project and see it through to the end, the results published.

The advice that I would give a nurse who may be considering such an endeavor is to "just do it." You will never be fully prepared for all the possible challenges along the way. That said, if you are fortunate enough to have a strong mentor, it could be the opportunity of a lifetime.

Another research study that I had the opportunity to participate in was a retrospective chart review to evaluate the relationship between neonatal hyperbilirubinemia and the use of oxytocics. In doing the retrospective chart review work, I learned firsthand how this type of research can answer questions related to best practice. I had the opportunity to present this research via poster abstracts at several conferences. Also, currently I am learning how to write a manuscript.

Acknowledgment: I'd like to extend my thanks to colleagues who have supported me throughout this whole process. In particular, I would like to thank Karen Gabel Speroni, Deena Lanham, Cindy Andrejasich, and the Research Committee.

Community Health Survey Research Study Evaluating Factors Linked to Breastfeeding Choices

Brigitte Taylor, RNC

Purpose: As specified by the Centers for Disease Control (CDC) in its *Guide to Breastfeeding Interventions*, protection, promotion, and support of breastfeeding are critical public health needs (U.S. Department of Health and Human Services, 2005). The Healthy People 2010 initiative set goals for increasing both breastfeeding initiation and duration. These goals include 75% of infants breastfeeding in the early postpartum period, 50% at six months, and 25% at 12 months. The Healthy People 2010 initiative also set goals to decrease disparities in these rates across all populations in the United States.

A variety of measures have been undertaken by Inova Loudoun Hospital (ILH) to support these goals, which include prenatal lactation classes, inpatient education by registered nurses, and lactation consultation per physician order. Also offered by ILH is a breastfeeding class that women can participate in without charge or preregistration requirements.

In 2004, there were approximately 2,109 deliveries, producing 2,124 births. From January 2005 to October 2005, there were 1,847 births. According to information obtained from a private consumer data tracking company, of 93 women surveyed, 71% breastfed their newborn while in the hospital, but only half indicated that they continued to breastfeed their infant at three months postpartum (one week = 61.3%; one month = 51.6%; two months = 34.4; and three months = 35.8%). These results were obtained from mothers who reside in the zip code areas that ILH serves. Currently, ILH does not maintain records on breastfeeding rates after discharge. Thus, it is difficult to ascertain if ILH is providing the most optimal community services, both prenatal and postpartum, to facilitate sustained high breastfeeding rates through 12 months postpartum. Therefore, a survey research study will be undertaken by ILH to determine these rates, the factors associated with the initial decision to breastfeed, and subsequent factors that result in continued breastfeeding or the decision to discontinue breastfeeding through 12 months postdelivery.

Design: This is a prospective survey research study on a convenience sample of women who birth babies at Inova Loudoun Hospital's Birthing Inn.

Methods: Once the informed consent process was completed and subjects provided signed informed consent, they were asked to complete the first study survey. Subjects were asked to complete the survey at follow-up time points of three, six, and 12 months postdelivery or until they were no longer breastfeeding.

Results: Enrollment for this study ended in December 2007. Data have not been analyzed. To date, approximately 300 subjects have been included in this study. Once all survey data have been received, methods of analysis, which will be descriptive in nature, will enumerate data on subjects who breastfeed their babies at birth and at the three intervals postpartum (i.e., three, six, and 12 months) during the first year of the baby's life. Descriptive statistics will be used for reporting study results and statistical comparisons (t tests, chi-square) to evaluate subjects who breastfeed through the first year of life and those who drop breastfeeding prior to that. These two groups will be compared by age, race/ethnicity, socioeconomic group, and other related breastfeeding factors as specified on the surveys. These groups will also be compared with the routine data collected for the general ILH population, including those who do not breastfeed at the time of hospital discharge. This includes, for example, race, age, labor type, if and how soon breastfeeding was attempted after delivery, the reason for not breastfeeding within one hour after delivery, patient type (e.g., private physician or clinic), infant gestation, primary discharge feeding type, and hospital length of stay.

Conclusions: This is an ongoing study. From an evidence-based practice perspective, the results from this study can be used by ILH to enhance existing measures to support initial decisions to breastfeed at the time of discharge, to develop new programs to support initial decisions to breastfeed at time of discharge, to enhance existing measures to support continued breastfeeding up to 12 months postdischarge, and/or to develop new programs to support continued breastfeeding up to 12 months postdischarge.

REFERENCES

U.S. Department of Health and Human Services. (2005). *The CDC Guide to Breastfeeding Interventions.* Retrieved November 17, 2008, from http://www.cdc.gov/breastfeeding/pdf/breastfeeding_interventions.pdf

CHAPTER 41

Yes, We'll Volunteer to Launch into Nursing Research

Gwen B. Phillips, Ruth M. Labardee, and Audrey Jones

It was a day like any other day in the life of a maternity department in a large tertiary care center in the Midwest. We had recently achieved Magnet status, and our leadership team was talking excitedly about nursing research involving the bedside nurses. As staff nurses, we had participated in studies initiated by physicians; however, we had no direct exposure to research by nurses for nursing. It sounded like an idea that was fresh, new, and interesting, and maybe a good resume builder. We raised our hands. "Sure," we offered, "we'll volunteer!" In answering the call, we did not realize what was in store for us.

The six weeks between the decision to embark on the research project and the first planning meeting were filled with questions. How could we do research? We didn't have any real knowledge about what was required. Wasn't research the pursuit of college professors? It sounded like something we were totally unqualified to do. We were staff nurses with decades of bedside experience, not white lab coat-clad scientists familiar with experimental techniques.

The more our team talked about nursing research, the more questions arose. What would the processes involve? Would we have enough time to make it happen, in addition to completing our normal work responsibilities? We were open to the idea of beginning nursing research within our department, but where would we start? What subject would we consider?

We held a series of meetings with staff nurses, advanced practice nurses, educators, the nursing department director, lactation specialists, and nurse managers. During one of our brainstorming sessions, a common topic of concern emerged: fluid intake during the intrapartum period and the effects on the mother and infant in the postpartum period. The lactation specialists and mother–baby nurses mentioned concerns about weight loss greater than 10% among some infants. What was the cause of this significant weight loss? Were these babies receiving adequate nutrition? Was successful breastfeeding being inhibited because of excessive maternal breast fullness from edema? Breast edema could make effective latch and suck difficult for the neonates. Were these babies losing weight in body mass from inadequate nutrition, or were they diuresing extra fluid received from their mothers prior to birth? Were the babies being given supplemental feedings beyond need?

Intravenous therapy is administered to all our patients. We were aware that the volume of fluid administered varied among patients, but we were not exactly sure by how much. Fluid administration practices varied among caregivers within the established protocols. As we sat around the table and began to talk about our individual practices of giving fluids during labor, we decided to review the records. We found fluid volumes routinely recorded on the anesthesia record of patients who had caesarean births; however, we could not always track the intake of patients with vaginal births. We were also frequently administering large amounts of fluid for other reasons without documenting the amounts. Exactly how much fluid was being given? More questions arose as we considered these issues. What was our current policy on recording intake and output for every laboring patient? What had been the experience of other clinicians? We started reviewing literature on fluid dynamics, changes in body composition, and infant weight loss. Our shared governance councils for nursing practice and research were consulted to help us prioritize the clinical questions.

Our quest to answer these and other questions became greater than any hesitancy to conduct research. As a result of our questions, discussions, and literature review, the purpose of our study was to examine and measure the relationship between the number of milliliters of fluid a mother receives in the intrapartum period and the impact on neonatal weight loss (measured in grams) and maternal breast fullness. It was an ambitious endeavor, but our sails were hoisted and we felt the breeze of favorable winds. We collected data for 248 mothers and their babies over the course of two months, and 200 qualified subjects were retained for the study.

After the study was completed, there were many feelings and thoughts running through our minds. First and foremost was the word *simplify*. We felt that we should have simplified our data elements—the number of data elements collected and the data collection tool. This was our first research study, and we wanted to be sure that we were collecting enough data to support our research questions. Instead of being so inclusive in our data, we should have been more specific and selective. We thought that perhaps if we collected an extra piece of data here and there, we would have data and ideas for future research. An extra meeting with our nurse researcher to narrow our data elements and tool would have been beneficial. Remember to keep it simple!

We felt we had to be captains of motivation for the rest of the staff throughout the study. At times it was difficult, but we all felt the need to keep the staff engaged. The extra work and time to collect data occasionally brought on feelings of frustration, apathy, and rejection among staff. Better staff preparation and involvement before the start of the project would have relieved the pressure and workload of the primary researchers. Some of us felt that dealing with negative staff feelings was one of the most difficult aspects of the study. We felt very excited, however, as we accomplished our goal and overcame the unknown of nursing research. It wasn't as hard as we thought it was going to be. Getting started is always the hardest part! It is exciting to think that our results may lead to significant changes in the care we provide our patients on a local and national level in the future. Overall, it was a wonderful learning experience! Yes, it was time consuming, but many hands made lighter work for all.

Hmmm, we're wondering what our next research project should be . . .

If you are wondering whether you are qualified to conduct research, let us assure you that you are! Cast off! The research waters can be turbulent, but you will get to the shore.

There are a few things we did that may help you overcome any apprehension you have about conducting research:

- Consult the experts. Our research team leaders were a research professor from the college of nursing and our clinical nurse specialist.
- Educate yourself. We took the time—and it did take time—to educate ourselves on several aspects of the research process using a tool required by our institution's research review board. It is a Web-based training program licensed by the Collaborative Institutional Training Initiative (CITI). The program provided a standardized approach to education on human subject research. It is easily accessible online at http://www.citiprogram.org.
- Expose yourself to research. We started attending the research journal club held once a month in our hospital. The articles are reviewed and analyzed for design, results, and significance. Attendance at the journal club meetings exposed us to the terminology of the research and made it less intimidating to start our project.
- If this is your first research project, choose a topic that is relevant and keep your clinical questions as focused as possible. Use simple tools and a simple process for data collection.
- Review literature about your topic and other research studies similar to the topic you are considering for study. Seek out hospital and community resources. Librarians are professionals at literature searches. Other nurses in your organization may be helpful advisors.
- Prepare the crew. Be sure that all know it's a big commitment. Members should represent all the nursing units involved in the study. Do everything you can to get the staff on your team before you begin data collection.

Announce the project using staff meetings, bulletin boards, and poster displays. Make sure the staff understand their roles and responsibilities. Recruit a large core group of staff participants to ensure success. You will also need nursing management's support of the research team's efforts in releasing staff for meetings and outlining staff participation expectations.
- Be enthusiastic, enjoy the voyage, and anchors aweigh!

The Relationship of Intrapartum Maternal Fluid Intake to Neonate Weight Loss and Maternal Breast Filling

Gwen B. Phillips, BSN, RNC; Ruth M. Labardee, BSN, RNC; and Audrey Jones, MSN, RN

Purpose: The purpose of this study was to examine relationships between the number of milliliters of fluids a mother receives in the intrapartum period, neonatal gram weight loss, and various factors related to the neonate and mother.

Design: A convenience sample of 200 subjects from a large midwestern acute care facility qualified for inclusion. Data were collected for the milliliters of intravenous and oral fluids administered to a mother from intrapartum admission to neonate birth. Neonate measurements included weight loss, 24-hour totals of urine and stools, and number of feedings. Maternal breast fullness was also measured.

Methods: This study used a nonexperimental research design with both multiple regression and descriptive statistics. Linear regression will be used to describe the relationships between these variables. Demographic information of both the mother and her neonate will be used to describe sample characteristics.

Results: Data analysis is pending. This study will assist nurses in predicting and addressing weight loss in neonates and breast fluid retention in mothers.

Conclusions: Findings from this research will enhance wellness-focused maternity practice and support optimal outcomes for the childbearing family. The study will provide valuable information on the relationship among the amount of intrapartum maternal fluids, neonatal weight loss, neonatal output, and various factors related to the mother and neonate. Findings will add to the general knowledge base on factors that contribute to neonatal weight loss and the amount of fluids women receive in the intrapartum period. Understanding patient demographics and in-hospital care events, nurses and lactation specialists can design primary interventions to predict and explain weight loss in neonates. Breastfeeding success can be enhanced if patients are in a supportive, informed care environment.

(Study design: January 2007–June 2007)
(Data collection: July 2007–August 2007)
(Data analysis: September 2007–March 2008)

CHAPTER 42

Taking the Long Road

Jeanne M. Rorke

Prior to doing our study, my only experience with nursing research was years ago during grad school. I was part of a group of students who implemented a study that looked at the influence of a breastfeeding class on breastfeeding duration. The experience was frustrating at the time because the members in my group had a difficult time getting together and following up on their work. Despite the frustration, I still dreamed of making a difference in the lives of our patients through research.

After several years of working in the neonatal intensive care unit (NICU), I was more passionate than ever about improving the outcomes of our tiny patients. I worked hard at research utilization, not having discovered evidence-based practice (EBP) at the time. The problem, I discovered, with research utilization is that there was not enough nursing research being done that could lend power to the conclusions. The evidence-based process is a fantastic way of looking at the evidence and systematically making decisions as to if, when, and how research findings can be used at the bedside. However, if there is not enough research going on about *nursing issues*, then we will not develop a body of knowledge to help us with our patients.

I decided to learn the process. Our neonatal fellows do research during their 2-year stay in the NICU. As part of the peripherally inserted central catheter (PICC) team (a team of nurses who insert and monitor peripherally inserted central catheters), we had many questions that we wanted answered. One of our questions was: Will trimming PICCs prior to insertion decrease catheter-related sepsis? At the time, it was standard practice in most NICUs to not trim the catheter prior to insertion. The PICC team felt that having too much catheter under the occlusive dressing contributed to loosening of the dressing, which in turn would lend itself to skin contamination near the insertion site. To make a long story short, one of the neonatal fellows and I did a study together. Although the PICC team and I did almost all the work, the fellow was the principal investigator and got most of the accolades for the study. The good news is that I learned the process of developing a well-designed study, writing an institutional review board (IRB) proposal and consent form, and many other aspects of the research process. I realized that I could do this process with a team of nurses.

Our unit formed a research/EBP committee. Our first meeting was spent brainstorming on all the nursing research questions that we had. We decided to do a very simple study that would make a big impact on our care. It was noted that our nasogastric and orogastric feeding tubes seemed to get dislodged frequently (they would fall out or get pulled out by the patient).This was so frustrating for the nurses who would have to get another tube and insert it. It was also hard on the babies because they ran the risk of aspiration, bradycardia, and stress when the tubes fell out or when we had to insert a new one. We knew that this topic would be a powerful motivator for the staff to participate in the data collection because of the impact of this problem on the babies and nurses. We used a simple design; it wasn't rocket science, but it worked for what we were trying to accomplish: a pre/post data collection period comparing our current method of securing feeding tubes with a new method that we had designed through talking to other hospitals and experimenting with different products. We were on our own for developing the new method because a thorough literature search found nothing on securing feeding tubes. We did find different methods in pediatric textbooks, but they were all based on opinion rather than research. The entire research project from conception to completion was about 10 months. Results showed that our new method was significantly better than our old method in preventing feeding tube dislodgement. The statistics were done by one of our neonatologists who supports nursing research. At the time, we did not have a statistics resource person in our hospital; now we do. I think that the statistics part of any research project is a daunting thought for budding researchers. Even our doctors have a statistician who advises them on what type of statistical tests should be used and then helps them with the actual statistics. Although this was not a large study, it was enough evidence for us to adopt the new method into practice.

I think that the most important thing to come out of this research project was that all the nursing staff participated in some way, by developing and writing the proposal, designing our new securement method, or participating in collecting the data. The staff saw that nursing research is not just for nursing professors or advanced practice nurses, but that there is a role for everyone. The research committee experienced a sense of pride in taking part in something that seemed to be out of our scope of abilities. All staff saw the benefit of participating in nursing research; it helped us to gain knowledge about discovering a different practice that ended up saving nursing time and being safer for the patient, and it ultimately saved money because fewer tubes were used.

My advice to new researchers is to start small; as you gain experience, you will learn. Choose a subject that will be of importance to the staff so that they will be motivated to participate with the project. Use your resources. Most hospitals have some types of resources: libraries, librarians, research nurse or consultant, clinical specialists, and/or nurses who have already had experience with research. Don't let the statistics get you down. Realize that we all need help with that area, so don't shy away. Share your results with others; we get lots of ideas from reading posters at conferences, articles in journals, and abstracts. Most of all, make it fun. Pick a small group of nurses who are excited about the process or learning the process. Celebrate your successes!

Comparison of Two Methods for Securing Nasogastric/Orogastric Feeding Tubes in the Neonatal Intensive Care Unit

Jeanne M. Rorke, MSN, RNC, NNP; Emily Randazzo, MSN, RNC;
Pamela Kilcullen, RN; Deborah Rosado, RNC, NNP; Julie Weiss, RN;
Elizabeth Froh, RN; and Judy Hanley, RN

Purpose: Feeding tubes are used frequently in the neonatal intensive care unit (NICU). Preterm infants and some full-term infants may have feeding tubes in for 30 days or more. Tubes can become dislodged by an infant for many reasons. Accidental feeding tube dislodgement can increase the infant's chances of vomiting and aspiration. More frequent feeding tube placements can result in increased stress to the neonate. The purpose of this study was to evaluate two different methods for securing feeding tubes in the NICU population.

Subjects: All infants admitted to our NICU who required nasogastric or orogastric feeding tubes were included. Neonates < 800 grams who were less than 2 weeks of age were excluded because of their fragile skin.

Design: This quasi-experimental design proceeded in two phases. In the first phase, data were collected for 8 weeks on all babies who had feeding tubes secured, using our standard method (op-site) to ascertain the rate of accidental feeding tube dislodgement. After the baseline data collection was completed, nursing staff were trained in a second method for feeding tube securement. This method required a different type of tape: abdominal retention tape. The tape was trialed on neonatal skin to assure that it was safe. In the second phase of the study, all patients eligible for the study had their feeding tubes secured with the new method. Data were collected for 8 weeks. The study was approved by the institutional review board at our facility.

Results: During Phase 1, the rate of accidental dislodgement was 25/100 feeding tube days (100 dislodgements in 390 feeding tube days). The rate during Phase 2 was 4/100 feeding tube days (26/670). The difference between

Phase 1 and Phase 2 was statistically significant using chi-square analysis: $p < 0.0001$ (CI = 95%, odds ratio = 0.13).

Limitations: Limitations of the study relate to the small size and the quasi-experimental nature of the research design. A larger, controlled study may yield different results. Sustainability of the positive results is an important factor in the evaluation of this project. Another data collection period is planned to occur 6 months after the new method is implemented.

Implications: The new method for securing nasogastric/orogastric feeding tubes resulted in significantly less accidental feeding tube dislodgements. Use of this method may result in less stress to the infant because of less frequent feeding tube dislodgements and increased placements. In addition, a decrease in feeding tube placements may result in a cost savings because fewer tubes are used.

CHAPTER 43

Big Ideas for Small Patients

Caryn Peters

Throughout my career in health care—all 29 years of it—I have gained quite a reputation for being the pain in the neck who would always ask "Why?" Never one to accept what is told to me at face value, I would always seek to understand the reasons for those actions. Still, it surprised me that I found myself applying for a nurse research position when it became available. After all, why would I desire to commit myself to a job that emanates from my most dreaded course as a student, that being nursing research?

But apply I did, and found myself in a new role for which I had no true training. I had earned the title of Neonatal Research Coordinator, and I now reported to the Director of Neonatal Research and Academic Affairs. Well, what's the big deal? It wasn't as if I had patients' lives at risk, right? And then it dawned on me like a boulder falling from the sky: I was responsible for this new, high-profile program, and the reputation of both the program and the internationally renowned physicians directing it rested on my shoulders. My naïve blundering could threaten both their integrity and credibility.

Getting back to my question of *why*, I was curious about new technology and how it could relate to neonatal intensive care. Pulse oximetry has become a standard of care in all aspects of medicine, especially in intensive care units. There has been an expansion of pulse oximetry to include measurements of perfusion, carboxyhemoglobin, and methemoglobin. Carboxyhemoglobin and methemoglobin previously have been measured through blood sampling only. The historic process is invasive and costly, and it requires special blood analyzers called co-oximeters. Thus, this new technology is called pulse co-oximetry.

Why would I even care about these values in a neonate? First, there are no established norms for this patient population, and I would have the chance to start that ball rolling and expand it to other centers if this is successful. Second, it is not well documented whether variables such as maternal smoking and environmental pollutants contribute to elevated blood levels of carbon monoxide. Third, elevated methemoglobin has been shown to be a precursor to sepsis, liver abnormalities, and hemolytic processes.

So, now I have a question: Where do I go from here? I validated the fact that the question has no current answer through a literature search. I had to go through the institutional review board (IRB) process for the first time, which seemed like a daunting task. As it turned out, I did more than what was needed by requesting a full review when it should have been submitted as an expedited review (lesson learned).

The use of a medical device in a study entails approval not only from the IRB but also from biomedical engineering, who requested yards of paperwork from the risk management department, the FDA, and the manufacturer. A pilot trial was performed on staff members. Those who were nonsmokers became upset by their high CO levels. It turned out that we had an outdated version of software that required an upgrade. Will the obstacles ever end?

On to the next stage, which consists of education for nurses in the neonatal intensive care unit (NICU), mother-baby unit, and labor and delivery. Cover letters were printed in English and Spanish so that nurses in all areas could submit information to family members about the likelihood that their baby could be enrolled in this noninvasive study. Privacy issues and assurance that all medical interventions would be consistent with routine care needed to be included with the information statements.

So, was it all worth it? I cannot give a complete answer until the study is completed in January 2009. I can tell you this: I probably looked like a complete fool when I was doing a little celebration dance in the NICU upon receiving my first-ever approval from the IRB. I'm also proud that I was able to work out all the little annoyances on my own, and I've gleaned a lot of lessons from it. Finally, I'm looking forward to results that could impact the practice of bedside clinicians around the world.

If I were to give advice to nurses who are contemplating research, I would tell them to seek out the resources that are available to them. The most important thing I've learned so far is to seek out allies and resources who have already done research and those who have done it within my own institution. Within my own neonatology group, I am lucky enough to have three individuals who are well published and knowledgeable in all aspects of research. Within the nursing realm at my hospital, we have a shared governance nursing research council chaired by the manager of nursing research who is doctorally trained. I was able to become a member of that committee and have been able to tap into her expertise on a regular basis. Another nurse researcher within the hospital has also proved to be invaluable as well. I also joined two research societies, the Association of Clinical Research Professionals and the Society of Clinical Research Associates, both of which have regular educational activities and journals that enhance my knowledge base. I thank them all for paving well-traveled roads for me to navigate on my journey.

Acknowledgment: I would like to extend my deep appreciation to all those in the MidAtlantic Neonatology Associates who believed in my ability to embark on the road to research, in particular Drs. Augusto Sola, Ben Lee, Marta Rogido, Andrew Schenkman, and Lawrence Skolnick, and, in addition, Patricia Vorel, Joanna Louie, and Dr. Susan Fowler, who have inspired and assisted me in my new role.

Normative Range of Values for Methemoglobin and Carboxyhemoglobin in Neonates Requiring Intensive Care

Caryn Peters, RNC, RRT

Purpose: The purpose of this study is to determine (1) the normative range of values for methemoglobin and carboxyhemoglobin in neonates requiring intensive care and (2) the correlation between pulse oximeter and blood values for methemoglobin and carboxyhemoglobin. Pulse oximeters provide vital information on the oxygen saturation in the blood without blood sampling or discomfort from needle sticks. This technology works by using photosensors that calculate an oxygen saturation value based on the light absorption of the blood detected when the pulsation of blood passes by. The calculated value is predicated on the assumption that the light is being absorbed by oxyhemoglobin, but in fact the receptor sites on the hemoglobin could be bound to carboxyhemoglobin or methemoglobin, which will affect the patient's ability to oxygenate. Many physiological, technological, and environmental factors can also affect the accuracy of the readings, including, but not limited to, carboxyhemoglobin, methemoglobin, fetal hemoglobin, light interference, intravascular dyes, electrocautery, hypotension, localized hypoxemia, sensor size or position, low oxygen saturation, sickle cell anemia, and sensor site temperature. Normal values for both methemoglobin and carboxyhemogoblin via pulse oximetry readings have not been established. The results of this study may reveal the need for modification of clinical guidelines for pulse oximetry in neonates.

Design: This is a descriptive correlation study not interfering with routine standard clinical care.

Methods: The sample includes all noninvasive measurement data obtained from infants who are on pulse oximetry (estimated sample size of 100: 25 in each of four different birth weight and gestational age categories). Comparisons will be made between the readings of the Masimo Rainbow signal extraction technology (SET) device and the actual measured blood values when possible. All blood measurement values used in the study will be from patients who already have indwelling arterial lines inserted for clinical indications, and the blood used will be from samples drawn for clinically indicated blood gas analysis. Data collected include the pulse oximetry readings and the correlating blood values of oxygen saturation, hemoglobin, methemoglobin, carboxyhemoglobin, and blood gas analysis. Readings from the Masimo pulse oximeter include perfusion index, pulse rate, carboxyhemoglobin, and methemoglobin, as well as oxygen saturation.

Analysis: Values will be compared to ascertain the accuracy of the pulse oximeter readings in relation to the blood values. Data for pulse oximetry will be obtained through Masimo Rainbow SET. Blood values will be analyzed by co-oximeters currently in use. Descriptive statistics will be performed on each variable, including means and standard deviations. Correlations will be made for each interval level data using the Pearson correlation statistic. Other statistics will be used as indicated.

Results and Conclusions: Pending.

CHAPTER 44

Warming Up to Research

Tina Daniels

Nursing is a profession that involves a lifetime of learning. I have been a neonatal intensive care nurse for 27 years. Phenomenal changes have occurred during this time, and for many years, I accepted those changes not really knowing or understanding where they came from. I began working on my bachelor of science degree in nursing, and my thirst for knowledge increased. I began attending conferences regularly. I applied for and obtained my RN3 on our clinical ladder. As an RN3, I was invited to participate in a group called Nursing Research Roundtable. This was my introduction to research and evidence-based practice.

I am very fortunate to be employed by Pinnacle Health System. The Nursing Research Roundtable comprises Pinnacle Health staff nurses, nurse educators, and senior nursing students from a nearby college. Together, in small groups, we set out to answer clinical questions through evidence-based practice and research. Our group consisted of our clinical nurse specialist, who acted as the group facilitator, our neonatal intensive care unit (NICU) staff development instructor, myself, and five nursing students. The first task at hand was to ask a "burning question."

We began to discuss certain aspects of neonatal care. Recently, two of our area hospitals merged. After this merging of two distinct NICUs, we found that the practice of thermoregulation in incubators was inconsistent. One facility used servo (skin) control until the infants were weaned to a crib. At the other facility, the infants were moved to air control for weeks before being weaned to a crib. Although these infants were able to maintain their temperature in air control, I always wondered if they were burning extra calories to do so. Did they gain weight more slowly on air control? Therefore, our Problem Intervention Comparison Outcome (PICO) question was: In neonatal infants in incubators/isolettes, what is the effect of servo control versus air control on their weight gain?

The next task at hand was our literature search. After an extensive literature search, we found that there was very little research on this subject. We found that keeping babies warm reduced neonatal death. We also discovered that babies' temperatures were more consistent in servo control than in air control, and incubator temperature was more consistent in air control than in servo control. There were no studies that measured weight gain in relation to thermoregulation. After critiquing the literature and reporting our findings to the research roundtable, we proposed to start a study in the NICU. I applied for and was granted the first research fellowship at Pinnacle Health System. This research fellowship provided me with a clinical nurse specialist as a mentor and 8 hours of paid time per month to work on my research project. This fellowship is offered only to staff nurses.

I was extremely surprised by the process of obtaining permission to conduct a research study. It was an incredible learning experience, and I now have a great respect for the process. The clinical nurse specialist, the staff development instructor, and I presented our proposal to the nursing research council, the hospital research committee, and the institutional review board (IRB). We had to ensure the safety of our participants. We completed education and training activities required by the IRB. All NICU staff were provided with education about research and evidence-based practice.

Prior to the start of my involvement in the research roundtable and my current research project, I was very intimidated by research. When I thought of the process of research, I imagined people in white coats working in a laboratory. I felt inadequate to participate in this type of academic exercise. I now feel inspired to find the best evidence to support my practice. I am empowered to remain at the bedside with my patients, enjoying my new expanded role.

Bedside nurses have the critical thinking skills necessary to ask the most relevant clinical questions. Seek the support you need to validate your practice. Do not be afraid to step out of the traditional role of the staff nurse. You have the potential to make the biggest difference by asking those questions and finding the answers. Utilize those people around you who can steer you onto the next step. One step at a time, you can continue to make health care better and better.

Acknowledgment: I'd like to extend my warmest thanks to colleagues who have helped to make this project possible. The following people have contributed their time and expertise to this project: Michalena Levenduski, MSN, RNC; Mary Lou Mortimer, RNC; Amy Helmuth, MS, RNC; Deborah Schafer, clinical nurse specialist; and Mary Kaye Flately, RD.

Thermoregulation: The Effect of Servo Control versus Air Control on the Weight Gain of Premature Infants in Incubators

Tina Daniels, RN, RNC

Problem Statement: The practice of maintaining thermoregulation for premature infants in our neonatal intensive care unit (NICU) and in NICUs around the world is very inconsistent. There are many differing opinions and approaches, with very little research to support practice. Providing a thermal environment that maintains a core temperature within a normal range is essential to the survival of a neonate. Thermoregulation is imperative also for optimal physiologic functioning. Currently there are two methods of thermoregulation in incubators, air temperature control and servo temperature control.

Purpose: The purpose of the study is to determine the effect of servo control versus air temperature control on weight gain in neonatal infants in incubators. With this study, we hope to determine and validate the best thermoregulation practice.

Design: This is a quantitative experimental study with a randomization of subjects. Random assignment will be accomplished through a computerized table of random numbers. The control group will be assigned to air temperature control, and the experimental group will be assigned to servo control. The independent variables will be the servo control and the air control in the incubator. The dependent variables will be the infants' axillary temperature and the infants' weight. All infants will have their axillary temperature maintained between 36.5 and 37 degrees C. Participation in the study will end when the infant has been placed into an open crib. There will be no difference in the quality of care. Consent will be obtained prior to inclusion.

Methods: A total of 250 neonates from 29 to 34 weeks gestation will be randomly assigned to either group. Neonates must maintain a temperature between 36.5 and 37 degrees C for 48 hours prior to inclusion. Exclusion criteria include neonates with congenital anomalies requiring surgical interventions and under phototherapy. Axillary temperatures and incubator temperatures will be measured and recorded every 3 hours. Neonates will be weighed daily between 1900 and 0700. Daily caloric requirements will be calculated. Subject withdrawal will occur if the subject is unable to meet caloric and protein goals for longer than 5 days.

Results and Conclusions: The study began on December 1, 2007. Preliminary data on 10 infants indicate that there is no statistically significant difference for weight gain or baby's temperature between the servo and the air control groups. Isolette temperature was significantly different in the air versus servo group. Data will continue to be collected, and t-test analysis will be used.

CHAPTER 45

Entering the Unknown Arena of Nursing Research

Maria Coussens and Donna Grochow

Before becoming involved in a study that looked at the effects of exercise on the growth and development of premature infants, our thoughts about research centered on the concept that research was designed and directed by physicians, and the nurse's role was very superficial. The concept of nurse-led research that involves the clinical nurse was not one that we had considered plausible. What could we do, as bedside nurses, that would be of interest to other clinicians? This all changed with the advent of the exercise study.

The last-trimester fetus typically demonstrates periods of physical activity through spontaneous movements against the uterine wall in a viscous amniotic environment, stimulating muscle mass and substantial bone strength. The infant born prematurely does not undergo this physical exercise "training" and often suffers from general growth impairment, inadequate muscle development, impaired neuromotor maturation, and poor bone formation (known as osteopenia of prematurity). The estimated rate of osteopenia in the infant < 1000 gm is 50%. It has been well documented that physical exercise is one of the most powerful stimulators of bone formation and growth, as well as muscle development. Therefore, a clinical trial of passive range-of-motion exercises was undertaken in the neonatal intensive care unit (NICU).

Nursing research is an exciting field with countless opportunities. The possibilities for potential nursing research topics are endless, and most of these topics are derived from the questions asked by the frontline nurse at the bedside. In my mind, research is now seen as a part of my responsibility, as a registered nurse, to bring evidence-based nursing to the forefront. All nurses, regardless of educational preparation, are qualified to participate in nursing research and can learn how to conduct quality research. Our small research study that started simply as a project for a nurse seeking advancement on the career ladder grew from a simple practice change, which was based on one small research study, to a randomized, controlled research study in a Level III NICU. From a small randomized controlled study, this research has now grown to a National Institutes of Health-funded 4-year study. The current study,

Assisted Exercise in Premature Infants: Effects and Mechanisms, has been funded by the National Institute of Nursing Research for $2.7 million. Current talks are centered on a future multicenter study that will expand on the current findings. It has been exciting to be involved in the growth of this study from a small nursing project to a potential multicenter study that could change the way premature infants are cared for across the nation.

Our advice to other nurses is to seek the opportunity to become involved in research. Find a mentor who can help you get started. Start by reading nursing journals that provide research articles. Read nursing journals that focus on your patient population or areas of interest to you. Ask questions. The frontline nurse has tremendous knowledge that pertains to the patient population whom he or she cares for. Bedside nurses have the opportunity to ask the questions that could potentially lead to better patient care. Frontline nurses often have questions but don't follow through with looking for the answers. Often, no answer exists, and there is no evidence that supports a certain nursing practice. This is the perfect starting point for a research question.

We have implemented the "sticky board" method to encourage frontline nurses to ask questions, find answers, and potentially develop research. The clinical investigation board, or sticky board, was developed in part after a review of the literature, which demonstrated a variety of effective methods to involve bedside clinicians in identifying potential clinical nursing research. The stick method is based on recommendations from the book *Research Strategies for Clinicians* (1999) by Granger and Chulay. Once posted, all staff members in the area are able to review the questions that prompt discussion. The answer to these questions may be addressed in an existing policy and procedure, may be administrative in nature, or may require nursing research. Members of the unit-specific practice council review the question, determine who will be responsible for each question, and post the answers. If no answer can be found, discussion can ensue on whether this is an area of interest for developing a research question.

Our last words of advice are really a recap: Don't be afraid of research, ask the questions that matter to your patients, and take a chance on making a difference!

Acknowledgment: The authors would like to acknowledge the expertise of neonatal clinical nurse specialist Robin Koeppel, MS, RNC; Dr. Dan Nemet; and Dr. Dan Cooper for the guidance, patience, and expertise they provided to us as novice researchers. We would also like to extend our warmest thanks to the director of the Department of Nursing Research and Education, Laura Bruzzone, MSN, RN, for her support and encouragement on our research journey.

The Effects of Exercise on Growth and Development in Premature Infants

Maria Coussens, RNC; and Donna Grochow, MS, RNC

Background: The premature infant is denied the most rapid period of growth and fetal development, which occurs naturally during the last trimester of pregnancy. Data collected from infants born at term demonstrated that this is the most crucial time for muscle and bone development and growth to occur as a result of the resistance provided by the uterus during fetal movement. Postnatal growth is dependent on the growth hormone (GH)→IGF-I axis. GH stimulates IGF-I through cellular GH receptors, the extracellular portion of which can be measured as GH binding protein (GHBP). Inflammatory cytokines such as IL-6 and IL-1ra can be elevated by stress or sepsis. IL-6 can inhibit GH→IGF-I activity. While IGF-1 levels and cytokines have been studied in neonates, their respective patterns in terms of neonatal growth have not been fully elucidated.

Hypothesis: Daily range of motion (ROM) exercises with gentle compression done on a premature infant in the neonatal intensive care unit (NICU) are believed to improve weight gain, increase bone density, and positively affect circulating levels of cytokines and growth factors.

Subjects: The UCI Institutional Review Board approved the study, and informed written consent was obtained. Fifty-eight premature infants (mean age 27.8 ± 0.4 gestational age) were enrolled into two study groups: Exercise and Control.

Methods: Subjects were enrolled into the study after becoming clinically stable and tolerating enteral feeds of 100 Kcal/Kg. Subjects were weighed and measured using calibrated scales and stadiometers at enrollment and on a weekly basis for the duration of the study. Bone Speed of Sound (SOS) was determined at enrollment and on a weekly basis for the duration of the study using the Sunlight Omnisense 7000S with the CS probe. Peripheral blood was collected via heel stick at baseline in weeks 2, 4, and 6 and at discharge and allowed to clot at 40oC. Serum was aliquoted and stored at $-80°C$ until assayed.

Results: Both the Exercise and Control Groups demonstrated similar patterns of bone SOS and changes in weight and length:

	Exercise (Before)	Exercise (After)	Control (Before)	Control (After)
SOS:	2884	2833	2995	2928
Weight:	1273	2386	1332	2441
Length:	37.5	44.8	39	45

The Exercise Group demonstrated a significantly more robust increase in GHBP and IGF-1 (Anabolic Mediator) and a significantly more robust decrease in IL-6 (Catabolic Mediator). Exercised infants had significantly higher levels of circulating IL-1ra at enrollment and discharge. IL-1ra showed a significant decrease in the exercise group from baseline (Catabolic Mediator).

Conclusions and Speculation: Unexpectedly, the bone SOS (density) response did not differ in the exercise group compared to the control group. Discharge weight and length parameters did not differ in the post-exercise group compared to the control group.

The circulating levels of GHBP and IGF-1 responded favorably to exercise compared to the response in the control group, and the circulating levels of IL-6 and IL-1ra responded favorably to exercise compared to the response in the control group.

The unexpected results pertaining to the bone SOS, weight, and length may be related to the timing of enrollment and the start of intervention. Previous studies have started the infants soon after birth. The average age of our infants was 4 weeks old at start of intervention. The unexpected results pertaining to the bone SOS, weight, and length may be related to the quality of the intervention. Previous studies have utilized one interventionist only. This study utilized the bedside nurse for the intervention.

CHAPTER 46

Project Preemie Research Recipe

Rosanna Welling, Laura Waszak, and Phyllis Lawlor-Klean

Ingredients:
2 cups of NICU RNs
2 heaping 8-hour training sessions
1 oz. NICU APN
1 oz. research RN
1 clove of subjects (117 tsp. NICU RNs, 18 Tbsp. PCAs, 7 medium neonatologists)
1 IRB application
1 INA application
2 amendments to IRB application

Directions:
Gather 2 eager NICU RNs to volunteer. Make sure RNs are sweet enough to blend together but tough enough to get through some of the other ingredients. Mix the RNs with the heaping training sessions. Boil the RNs with lots of new evidence-based information. Then knead the new information with the APN. Grease the IRB and INA applications with light oil. Place 2 amendments to the IRB application on the side to add later. Next, preheat the oven to 142 degrees of surveys. Whisk up a standardized educational protocol and spread it evenly over subjects. Place in oven and bake for 18 education classes for staff to attend. Before removing from oven, poke holes with pre- and posttests to determine if subjects need more education. Sprinkle the amendments on top. For a rich and creamy taste, clarify with the research RN over this entire recipe.

Standardization of an Educational Feeding Program for All Preterm Infant Caregivers

Rosanna Welling, MBA, RN; Laura Waszak, RN; and
Phyllis Lawlor-Klean, MS, RNC, APN/CNS

Background: Adaptation to different feeding techniques among clinicians in the neonatal intensive care unit (NICU) can be difficult for preterm infants. Infants are often discharged before mastering oral feeding skills. Clinicians are not aware of infants' readiness to oral feed or the proper support and feeding techniques for adequate nutrition and growth.

Purpose: Our challenge was to develop and implement a standardized educational feeding program for all preterm infant caregivers. The program emphasized infant readiness, consistent oral feeding techniques, a common language between clinicians, and instruction for parents.

Method: During this phase, the NICU staff's knowledge of the premature infant's readiness to feed and current feeding practice were evaluated. A validated oral feeding survey was distributed to all NICU staff, and consent was implied by survey completion. Descriptive analysis was used to determine variance from evidence-based neonatal feeding readiness practice.

Results: Subjects were 117 nurses, 18 patient care assistants, and 7 neonatologists. Findings showed that many inconsistencies exist among the staff about the indicators used to initiate oral feedings. Approximately 41% of staff were not assessing for signs of feeding readiness, using gestational age or other indicator before feeding. The behavioral characteristic reported as used "almost all the time" by 59% of nurses was observed sucking.

Conclusions: Oral feedings should not be based simply on gestational age but on assessment of signs of readiness. To facilitate staff learning needs and effect change in practice, assessment of current knowledge was important prior to the development of a practice change.

CHAPTER 47

Exploring New Possibilities and How It Can Change Your Practice and Your Life

Renee Houser

I received my LPN diploma in June 1989. This memorable day was also my first day of orientation at the Penn State Milton S. Hershey Medical Center. In the 18 1/2 years of being a nurse, I have worked in two areas. The first 8 1/2 years, I worked on a medical-surgical floor, where I mainly took care of post-operative patients who had coronary artery bypass surgery. I now work in the outpatient allergy, asthma, and immunology clinic. Like most people, I am comfortable with familiarity. I enjoy my job and know what is expected of me and how to accomplish it. The thought of change and being taken out of my comfort zone is scary. However, I have learned how rewarding it can be to have the courage to open the door and step out into the unknown.

My venture into the unknown began approximately two years ago. One of my daily duties was administration of allergy injections. I would do all the required steps in medication administration. First I would check the schedule to see who was coming for his or her injections, pull the chart, check the dose that the patient was scheduled to receive, draw it up in a syringe, and label it on a tray. There were times when patients would need to reschedule their visits or have dose changes because of a reaction from a previous injection. Charting would generally be completed after the session had ended.

There were too many stumbling blocks regarding how things were being carried out. Sometimes extract-filled syringes were being thrown away because patients did not show up for their appointment. There was also the risk of giving the patient the wrong drug or an incorrect dose of the correct drug. The potential for inconsistent and incomplete labeling, incomplete charting, and lack of patient identifiers were some of our concerns. Providing allergy injections is a large-volume practice; we knew there had to be a better way to ensure that the process was being carried out safely. We needed to find out what it was! How did other allergy practices handle this type of situation?

One day, one of our physicians who is a visiting professor told us of an electronic program he had recently purchased. Our interest was piqued; could this be what we were looking for? My coworkers and I wanted to know more. What did this program have to offer, and would it resolve our concerns? Following our inquiry, we learned that an electronic program not only would decrease the risk of human error but also could also make our practice more efficient. The program labels the vials with barcodes to ensure correct patient and vial strength, with easy access to document reactions. The patient's history of injections is accessible by only a mouse click, and all adverse reactions are displayed and highlighted in red. Other benefits include an "alert" section for notification of vial expiration dates, a section to order new serum vials, a mixing screen to provide accuracy, and printed labels that are patient-specific, to name a few. Wow! How cool is this?

We then took the next step: convincing the allergy, asthma, and immunology chief physician and our office manager that this program was a worthwhile purchase for us. We explained the benefits of the program, those that would lead to greatly increased patient safety. We also explained how this would improve patient care outcomes and satisfaction. The five nursing "rights" of medication administration were made especially visible in this system: right patient, right route, right time, right medication, and right dose. Equipped with the best available evidence, we received an affirmative Yes! It was official. We were going to purchase the program and would be the first "training program" to have it.

In the spring of 2005, we found ourselves making a road trip to Altoona, Pennsylvania, where we would learn how to use the program. What a day; there was so much to learn. An employee at the corporate office answered our questions and gave us great hands-on practice to familiarize us with how the program works. At the end of the day, we left with a manual of all the things we learned—and also with a sense of bewilderment about how we were going to get the program up and running.

With the dedication and determination of all of us, we started by entering the demographics and allergy orders for over 200 patients. During this time, we began to educate the patients about the program and the changes that they would soon be encountering. We emphasized the benefits of increased safety and efficiency. The day finally came in August 2005: The program was ready to go live. It was a day of feeling nervous, excited, and scared all wrapped into one. We demonstrated how the system worked to all interested patients, hoping that they would be just as excited as we were to be using it at last. Some of them did not care for the amount of time it took, but we reassured them that given a little time, everyone would become more familiar with the program. Once this adjustment occurred, it would make everything easier and more efficient. However, like everything in life, there are stumbling blocks, and we ran into a few. In no time at all, our questions and problems were resolved with help from the technical support team at the corporate headquarters. It was certainly worth all the time and energy it took to enter the data needed.

Given the challenges we had and the successes that we eventually achieved, a physician at one of our staff meetings suggested that the nurses submit a poster about the electronic program for the annual conference held by the American Academy of Allergy, Asthma & Immunology. The conference was going to be held in Miami, Florida. Without giving it much thought, I said yes, I would give it a try. I asked my coworkers if they wanted to help. We had never done anything like this before. Our first question was, How do we get started? With guidance from two physician mentors and a lot of writing and rewriting, we composed our first abstract. I submitted the abstract entitled "Modern Technology Making Immunotherapy Safer" in September 2005. The waiting that followed was the hardest part. Would the abstract be accepted?

On December 7, 2005, I received the e-mail that we were waiting for: Our abstract was accepted! How exciting! Then, more good news: Our abstract was also being considered for a travel grant. Wow! Could this really be happening to such novices? The next task was to turn the abstract into a poster. Our mentors came to our rescue with suggestions and ideas on how to accomplish this. We considered different ideas and finally came up with a plan for visuals to place on the poster. We were able to obtain screen shots of the system directly from the program. I had taken a picture of a coworker using the card scanner and a picture of another coworker to show one of the patient identifiers. Finally, things were starting to come together, and I was having a lot of fun. After we had everything together on a PowerPoint presentation, it was sent to strategic services, where it became a poster. I received a letter in January stating, "On behalf of the Education and Research Trust (ERT) of the American Academy of Allergy, Asthma & Immunology (AAAAI), I am writing to congratulate you on being chosen as the recipient of the 2006 ERT Allied Health Travel Grant Award." The letter also mentioned that this specific travel grant is given to the top three abstracts submitted for the AAAAI annual meeting. The abstract would also be published in the annual meeting final program, and the award recipients would be acknowledged in the membership newsletter, "The Academy News." A special benefit dinner would be held, where I would be asked to step on stage with other winners to receive the award. I was stunned; I had never experienced anything like this before. I couldn't believe this was really happening.

We traveled to Miami, where we proudly presented our poster and answered questions from other conference attendees about the program. Upon returning from our adventure, we hung the poster in the clinic for all to see. Back to reality and to a regular work day. But wait, there is more to come. Our outpatient nurse educator and our professional practice nurse leader heard about the poster and came to see it for themselves. They suggested that I enter the poster in the Department of Nursing's Nancy R. Kruger Award for Clinical Scholarship. This award is given each year during the nurses' week celebration. We found ourselves once again named as award recipients. We had our picture taken with the chief nursing officer; we received flowers and a check; and we were acknowledged in the systemwide newsletter, *The Crescent*. I felt very proud to be a part of this honor and recognition as I received congratulations from my colleagues. Once the word spread about the program that we were using in our clinic, the outpatient pediatric allergy clinic became interested as well. We were more than happy to show them how the system worked. After stressing the evidence showing increased safety to the patients, they too were intrigued with the program and have since had it installed.

Work had once again returned to normal until our nurse educator approached me with a question. Where was the information kept on how to complete specific procedures that were done in the allergy clinic? I looked at her and pointed to my head—that's where they were. She suggested that I write down the procedures and place them in a manual. This type of manual would be beneficial to both the nursing staff and to the allergy fellows. I didn't realize how many procedures we do that are specific to our clinic until I started making a list—skin testing, medication testing, mixing allergy serum, administration of allergy injections, and conducting spirometry tests, to name a few. Boy, did I have a lot of work to do. With guidance and help from the section chief and the professional practice nurse leader, I was able to meet this challenge. The procedures, based on evidenced-based best practices, were completed and then taken to the outpatient practice council. This council is one of three outpatient councils that were developed as part of our Magnet journey, and it is now one of the working councils in the shared governance structure of the Department of Nursing. The allergy clinic was the first outpatient clinic to obtain approval from the council for clinic-specific procedures. The outpatient quality of work life is another council developed on our Magnet journey. I have been a member of this council since it was first developed and now hold the honor of being chair of the council.

Little did I realize that the Magnet journey that everyone at Penn State Hershey Medical Center was experiencing would eventually be such a large part of my life as a nurse. The journey, from the initial work that my colleagues and I did to show our evidence-based practices to participation in shared governance, was exciting in and of itself. I was privileged to volunteer for, and be selected as, a room monitor for the Magnet site visit. I was intrigued because I enjoyed listening to other colleagues talk about their experiences. That was the easy part (listening and learning), but the Magnet site appraisers wanted to visit the allergy clinic. The thought made me nervous and excited at the same time. I did my best to answer their questions and then started talking about the clinic's electronic system for allergy injections and how it increased patient safety. The next day I received a phone call. The site appraiser was very impressed with the program and requested additional information to share this evidence-based practice with other facilities.

What a great experience the journey to receiving Magnet status turned out to be for all of us. I still find it amazing how many doors have opened since I first had the courage to step into unfamiliar territory. I am looking forward to participating in the future plans that the Department of Nursing has for developing a LPN clinical ladder. After that, who knows? There are endless possibilities, including pursuit of further education as a registered nurse. The past 2 years have been the most rewarding and exciting years of my nursing career thus far. I am eager to see what is behind the next door and where it will take me. I challenge all who read this story to take that step and see how exciting and rewarding it can be. I hope you receive as much satisfaction in your work as I have in mine.

Acknowledgment: I would like to acknowledge and thank the following people: Ruth Gundermann, BSN, RN, professional practice nurse leader, and Claudette Beamesderfer, MS, RN, clinical nurse educator, for the support and encouragement they gave me to open the doors and step into unfamiliar territory; coworkers Jennifer Hunter, medical assistant, and Stacey Shaeffer, LPN, for helping to find a way to improve the safety in the administration of allergy shots, for their dedication in helping to implement the program, and for all their help in making our first poster such a success; Laura Fisher, MD, and Timothy Craig, DO, for their support, knowledge, and expertise; and Jeffrey Rosch, MD, and Lee Johnson, employees of Rosch Visionary, for helping us.

Modern Technology Making Immunotherapy Safer

Renee Houser, LPN, Lead Clinic Nurse

Rationale: A recent trend in allergy has been standardization to decrease the risk associated with skin testing and immunotherapy. Electronic programs further help in decreasing errors by practice standardization, charting, and obliged queries.

Design: Human error accounts for a significant number of mistakes associated with administration of allergy vaccine. Standardization and an electronic program were recognized as ways to decrease errors.

Methods: Computerized immunotherapy with personalized scan cards was instituted in the spring of 2005. After the patient's card is scanned, the immunotherapy records are visualized along with the patient's picture. A printed label on each vial allows the scanner to verify that the vial is the appropriate strength for that specific individual. The electronic program shows the previous dose and when it was given. It then prompts for the next scheduled dose to be given. All adverse reactions from previous injections are highlighted in red. After the injection is given, a built-in timer monitors the length of time the patient is observed before charting the results. The program prompts for peak flow and designates peak flow values to hold immunotherapy.

Results: Review of the literature of immunotherapy indicates that most errors are clerical and due to inappropriate doses or to patients receiving incorrect extracts. Each error is addressed with the electronic immunotherapy program, therefore decreasing the risk associated with immunotherapy. Electronic immunotherapy has been effective in our office in improving quality of care.

Conclusion: With the help of an electronic program and using the "five rights"—right medication, right dose, right time, right route, and right patient—immunotherapy administration is now safer.

(2005)

CHAPTER 48

From Problem to Project to Publication

Peggy Malone

It wasn't rocket science; it was a problem we nurses knew in our gut needed fixing. It wasn't vast knowledge about the significance of p values; it was listening to remarks from satisfied patients that prompted a survey. In nursing, research sometimes finds *you*—be ready to grab it and take a shot at publishing your work. The endeavor will fill you with feelings of pride and power.

As a unit-based, or "floor," nurse, the idea of research seemed out of my league. I mistakenly assumed that research was conducted by PhD-prepared persons in fancy suits or "silk-blouse nurses," as they are colloquially known. I never thought a bedpan-toting, elastic-waisted, scrub-pants-wearing nurse could get her name in print. But I did!

My study was prompted when chemotherapy nurses in our cancer clinic began to have a discussion during lunch break about the long-known difficulties arising from high anxiety levels of first-time chemo patients. An oft-heard refrain in our break room was, "I felt so sorry for my patient today; he/she was really scared."

Our clinical nurse specialist overheard our talk and told us about a new project at the main hospital. The orthopedic department was conducting presurgery teaching on their total knee patients. These patients, armed with knowledge before the actual surgery, appeared to the orthopedic nurses to be less overwhelmed and more compliant after discharge. That was all we nurses needed to hear—the seed was planted. Soon we were off and running with our own patient teaching project!

A literature search was done, a task force was formed, and our clinical nurse specialist devised a PowerPoint presentation. We began enrolling first-time chemotherapy patients in the 1-hour chemo class, which was facilitated by a rotation of staff nurses, all of whom were oncology certified.

As time passed, more and more patients attended the classes. The chemotherapy nurses heard positive comments from patients about the class and recognized behavioral differences from the chemotherapy class "graduates."

The patients and families were calmer, had fewer questions, and retained information about the medications better. In addition, remarks from patients and families *during* chemotherapy class were indicating enthusiasm for the teaching format. Comments included, "This class was powerful," "I am so grateful I could sit down and talk about this before I actually started treatment," and "My daughter was happy she could come and hear about what I will be going through."

We decided to measure customer satisfaction scientifically. We developed a survey with Likert scale measurements and mailed them to patients in a self-addressed stamped envelope. The data revealed high satisfaction among our patients and their families with the chemotherapy class (see the abstract).

In an effort to pass on this valuable information, my manager suggested that we develop a poster project for a local nursing symposium event. My abstract was accepted, and the poster presentation ended up taking first place at the symposium! I was elated and then submitted to our hospital newsletter the information from my poster session in article form.

The spark that moved me on to publication came from my clinical nurse specialist, who said to me of the study results, "This is publishable." My little nurse-heart soared at hearing those words, and once I heard them, there was no giving up on my part.

It was a good thing I had such strong feelings about the value of my study because I had to persevere. I made revisions and looked up several more articles to add veracity to my study. I submitted, revised, resubmitted. Each step of the way, my mentor was with me handing out words of encouragement: "You can do this!"

The entire experience was beyond exciting. I was enlightened on several fronts, like learning the difference between the words *emend* and *amend*, and how to make those little bar graphs in the Excel computer program. Best of all, I learned I could be conversant about research and sophisticated in my writing. Nurses have vast amounts of insight on a multitude of topics. I truly believe that once a nurse begins expressing what has been learned from experiences at the bedside, the depth of knowledge harbored within shocks even us.

The day the journal arrived in the mail with my published article, I immediately brought a copy to my mom's house. She said, "Sweetheart, I don't understand one word of this thing except your name, but I'm sure it is a wonderful article." My mom went on to say that she was never so proud of me and was sorry that my dad was not alive to see that one of the kids had (in Dad's words) "done good."

I think of the three H's when advising anyone on doing research.

1. *Hear the milieu.* Keep your ears perked for events happening on your unit. What are your coworkers talking about? Good and bad. What do the patients and families say? Nearly anything has merit as a potential study.
2. *Hang in there.* Patience is a virtue when you go from problem to publication. The process takes time to develop. Be open with both yourself and the journal to which you are submitting. Don't give up. As soon as you get suggestions for revisions, sit down and work on them. Keep your eyes on the prize.
3. *Heroes.* Look to your heroes in the workplace with advanced degrees or to those who have published before. They know what you need to do to stay on track. They know how publishers think. Share the ups and downs with them. Your heroes will be as excited as you are during the process.

I'm not afraid of p values anymore. My attitude about research is now one of embracement. Nurses in the midst of patient care *should* be the people conducting research. We have the elements of change within our grasp because of both our desire to do the best for our patients and the art of intuiting a better way.

My hospital put out a press release when my article appeared in the journal. Many of my nurse colleagues congratulated me, and to each I responded, "Thank you. *You* are next." And I meant it. We are *all* nurse researchers, and we all have the expertise for proving better patient care right in our nurse "noodles"—so get out there and get going because, *you* are next.

Acknowledgments: The author would like to acknowledge the expertise of clinical nurse specialist Judy Williamson for her humor, guidance, and patience during my novice research journey.

Patient Satisfaction with Chemotherapy Education Class

Peggy Malone, BS, RN, OCN, OSF

Purpose: The Center for Cancer Care has traditionally provided outpatient chemotherapy teaching in the clinical setting while the patient receives his or her first treatment. Patients were anxious on that first chemotherapy day, and retention of information was lacking. Based on a literature review, the idea for doing patient/family education in a group setting was presented to the nursing staff, who then helped develop the format. The Chemotherapy Education Class project was an oncology-certified nursing-facilitated 1-hour class for patients and families prior to their first treatment, followed by a survey to measure the satisfaction of this format.

Design: A survey was created to measure patient/family satisfaction with chemotherapy class using a Likert scale rating.

Methods: Patients undergoing chemotherapy for the first time were referred by the physician or nurse to the chemotherapy class prior to their first chemotherapy treatment. Classes were held in the cancer center library and facilitated by an oncology-certified nurse, using a standardized educational format. A patient satisfaction survey was mailed to participants after they had received several treatments in their course. The survey included eight questions, rated on a Likert scale, which focused on the effectiveness of the class. Space for comments and suggestions was included. Twenty-eight surveys were distributed.

Results: A 60% response rate revealed *good* to *excellent* in 84% of the survey responses. All comments included were favorable. In addition, 16% of responses focused on the desire for more detailed information.

Conclusions: Educating patients prior to their first chemotherapy experience may help to improve their ability to cope. After a diagnosis of cancer, patients and families experience a significant need for information about treatment and side effects. Improved coping strategies may result from nurses meeting with patients and families in a quiet environment prior to the start of treatment.

CHAPTER 49

Research Can Be Fun and Interesting

Gail Probst

I completed graduate school almost 20 years ago. Fourteen years after I received my bachelor of science degree in nursing, I thought it was time to get my master's. My rationale for having my master's in nursing was that it would increase my knowledge base and lead to promotional opportunities. Not unlike many young women who finished their undergraduate degree in their early 20s, I was 34, had four children, held a part-time job at a hospital 40 minutes from my home, and was very busy with life.

I remember that I struggled with going to graduate school and managing my family. There were too many commitments and so little time. More than once, I considered ending my graduate education before I finished. Research and writing a thesis frightened me, and I tried to block the thought of the whole project.

School went well even with my four children and their constant school and social activities. I received my master's degree in nursing 4 years after I began. It truly was a milestone for me. Research, on the other hand, remained a constant and frightening challenge during my years in graduate school. I was convinced that nursing research had no relevance to my everyday practice. I took the nursing research core course and learned such terms as *theoretical framework, randomization, null hypothesis*, and *deduction*. How could this new language really help me in my nursing practice?

I remember thinking that advanced practice nurses should excel in administration, education, clinical practice, and research. I knew I had a fairly good handle on nursing education and administration and was proficient in my clinical skills, but I had no confidence at all in my research skills. Now, could I just get a passing grade on my research project and be done with research? My thoughts about research became more discouraging, especially when I had to write my thesis. I never felt good about "composition writing," as it was called in my English class in the 1960s. I had to write my thesis several times to get it just right. I knew my topic was timely and relevant to nursing. My research question was: Would providing education on death and dying better prepare nurses to care for patients who are dying? Even I would admit that at the end of the thesis process, my bound finished thesis was very impressive! More important, I felt better about this "research dimension" of the advanced practice nurse role. To this day, my thesis sits on my bookshelf at home and in the library of the school of nursing, and I am very proud of this accomplishment!

Now, 20 years later, my experience has continued to be improved with my clinical skills, and educational and administration abilities. I now realize the value of nursing research. Nursing has moved from tradition based to evidence based, and I want to be part of the movement that advances nursing science.

I have been working in oncology nursing for over 18 years, and I just love the work I do. I do an extensive amount of work with women who have breast cancer. I provide a consultation service and preoperative teaching to patients and their significant others. I have facilitated a breast cancer support group twice a month for the last 15 years.

Because I do so much consultative work with women who have been diagnosed with breast cancer, I have observed that if nurses educate and support the partners of women with breast cancer, the whole family will get through the illness in a cohesive manner and experience less anxiety and better marital satisfaction.

Coincidentally, while I was considering the hypothesis, "When partners of women with breast cancer receive education and support, the couple will experience less anxiety and achieve better marital satisfaction," I received a grant from the New York State Department of Health to facilitate support groups especially targeting partners and children of women with breast cancer.

Now was the perfect time to get into nursing research. With some encouragement and help from the assistant director of nursing and coordinator of nursing research/evidence-based practice at Huntington Hospital, I embarked on my first real nursing research project.

I have been through the entire research process now and have to admit that it was extremely interesting and educational. I had the opportunity to speak with a psychologist from Canada who had the same research interest in women with breast cancer and their partners. I can now write an abstract, do a review of the literature, define my methodology, present my research to the institutional review board, speak to other researchers about my findings, and use the language of research. I also admit that I remain a research novice but know that if I have the time in my busy day, I would love to spend more time researching topics in cancer care.

For those nurses considering nursing research, I would encourage them to start small, but start. Once you have done nursing research once or twice, you will understand the language and the process. You will understand what you are able to accomplish within a specified time frame. Pick topics that interest you, and search out a nurse who is comfortable in nursing research and then let him or her guide you.

Once I had decided what my topic would be, it came together very nicely and really didn't take very much time. Initially I was disappointed that I didn't get the required number of subjects to participate in my study. However, I learned a great deal of valuable information regarding the research process that will be of great value to me in my future research endeavors.

Acknowledgment: I would like to thank Dr. Judith Moran-Peters, whose gentle, friendly, persistent guidance convinced me that the only way to manage the information and my observations with the grant I received was to incorporate research into my practice. Her guidance, never overwhelming, let me develop insight into the research process and develop new skills (after so many years as a RN) while having fun at the same time.

Evaluation of the Effectiveness of Specific Interventions on Spouses of Women with Breast Cancer

Gail Probst, MS, RN, CNA, ANP, OCN, AOCN, BC

Purpose: To evaluate the effectiveness of specific interventions on spouses of women with breast cancer.

Design: This institutional review board-approved descriptive study was designed to gather information for the development (including a formal power analysis) of a randomized trial examining the effect of education and support intervention on the mood and marital satisfaction experienced by the spouses of women with breast cancer.

Method: The sample consisted of 5 women diagnosed with Stage I, II, or III breast cancer, and their spouses. Spouses were defined as the married male partner of a woman with breast cancer. Interventions for the spouse included two educational sessions taught by a registered nurse and a medical oncologist. The educational sessions were followed by four sessions of a support/intervention group 1 week apart for spouses, facilitated by an oncology nurse and a certified social worker. The study evaluated the mood changes of the patient and spouse as measured by the Profile of Mood States (POMS) and the marital satisfaction as measured by the Index of Marital Satisfaction (IMS). The patient and the spouse completed the pre- and posttest, but education and support were provided only to the spouses.

Results: No significant difference was found between the pre- and posttest for the POMS and IMS for the patients and their spouses.

Conclusions: This study provided important information concerning women with breast cancer and their spouses. Healthcare professionals should consider providing education and support to the patient and her spouse from the time of initial diagnosis through the treatment phase. Support and education should be provided to both the patient and her spouse together rather than as separate entities.

CHAPTER 50

Research: Quaking in My Boots

Butch O. Blake

When my boss asked me to take over a research project she was trying to get off the ground, I thought she had lost her mind. Me doing research? She didn't know what she was asking. I didn't have the slightest clue how to take on this task. And PICOT, what is that? Isn't it some type of coat you wear when it's cold? But when my boss sat down with me and explained that very little research was done involving orthopedic surgical patients and how much these patients would benefit from my expertise, I reluctantly said okay. My boss explained to me about wanting to know if there was a problem with patients coming into the operating room for surgery and having elevated blood sugars. Did the patient know it? What effect did increased blood sugars have on post-operative infections? I was totally hooked. With the help of my boss and coworkers, I started educating myself about nursing research. What I thought was a daunting task really wasn't so bad once I broke it down. I handled things the best I could on my own and then asked for help with things I knew little or nothing about. I tackled this idea with the same enthusiasm and drive as with everything in my life, and boy did it pay off. One of the best feelings is when you start your research project and start seeing your labor bear fruit; it's very gratifying! I guess the best thing about doing research is the knowledge you gain, and then being able to put that knowledge toward helping improve patients' well-being. That's what it's all about—taking care of our patients. If you're afraid of the word *research*, don't be. There are tons of resources out there to help make doing research easier. My best advice to you is to find a good mentor, someone who has experience in research and who can guide you on the right path to research greatness! Finally, just let me say that I'm not quaking in my boots anymore, and I now know what PICOT means! It is an acronym used to help identify clinical questions: P = patient/problem/population; I = intervention; C = comparison; O = outcome; and T = time. I'm not quaking in my boots!

Identification of Blood Glucose Trends Intraoperatively in Patients Undergoing Major Joint Replacement Surgery

Butch O. Blake, ADN, RN

Clinicians face the challenge of minimizing adverse clinical outcomes for patients who undergo invasive surgical procedures. In the case of orthopedic surgical patients who undergo major joint replacement, a surgical site infection can be catastrophic clinically, emotionally, and financially. It has been well documented that poor blood glucose control is a major risk factor for surgical site infections (Streeter & Haley, 2006). In addition, poor blood glucose control increases patients' mortality risks. One study examined 2,030 patient medical records and found that the stress of new hyperglycemia was associated with higher in-hospital mortality rates (16%) compared with those patients with a prior history of diabetes (3%) and subjects with normoglycemia (1.7%). The preponderance of research examining the effects of poor blood glucose has focused on the intensive care unit (ICU) and cardiac surgery populations. In another study, coronary artery bypass patients with an average glucose level above 250 mg/dl had a 14.5% mortality, compared with 0.9% in patients with glucose levels below 150 mg/dl. Normal blood glucose is considered 80–110 mg/dl (Van den Berghe et al., 2006).

No determination has been made of the extent of the effect of poor glycemic control on the mortality or complication rates among orthopedic surgical patients. Studies examining the prevalence of poor glycemic control during orthopedic patients' perioperative course are nonexistent. Mraovic et al. (2006) conducted a study involving a cohort of orthopedic surgical patients over a 2-year period to assess healthcare providers' blood glucose management. The researchers found that glucose control was poor. Only 8% of patients had their glucose levels treated or adjusted, and standard glucose monitoring was not performed in 86% of the patients studied.

Despite evidence showing that insulin protocols for controlling intraoperative glucose levels are successful in managing the cardiac surgical patient, such evidence is not available for the orthopedic surgical population. Research is needed to understand the prevalence of the problem and the effects of poor blood glucose control before attempting to initiate similar protocols in orthopedic surgery. This study is a preliminary study designed to identify the extent to which abnormal glucose levels exist among orthopedic patients preoperatively and intraoperatively. Findings will determine the potential for abnormal glucose control to be a risk factor in the orthopedic surgical population.

RESEARCH QUESTIONS

1. What proportion of orthopedic patients undergoing major joint replacement surgery present on the day of surgery with blood glucose levels above 110mg/dl?
2. What proportion of patients undergoing major joint replacement surgery experience elevated blood glucose levels intraoperatively above 110mg/dl?
3. What is the relationship between patient demographics and the incidence of elevated blood glucose levels? Pearson's correlation will be used to determine if there is a relationship between patient demographics and elevated blood glucose levels.

Design: This proposal is for a descriptive pilot study. A convenience sample of adult orthopedic surgical patients undergoing first-time elective major orthopedic joint replacement surgery will be enrolled in this study. We are projecting 100 patients for enrollment. Patients excluded from the study will be those having urgent/emergent major joint procedures added to the orthopedic operating room schedule on the day of surgery, and major joint revision patients, who are more likely to have had a previous wound or joint infection.

Method: When patients enter the perioperative holding area, a member of the research team will approach eligible patients to explain the purpose of the study and obtain written consent. Patients who agree to participate in the study will receive a bedside capillary glucometer test in the holding area. The bedside capillary glucometer test is an invasive procedure that is standard for monitoring blood glucose levels. This test requires a finger puncture with a sterile lancet to obtain less than 1 ml of blood for testing. With the use of standard antiseptic techniques, the risk of infection following the finger puncture is very low. The researchers will also collect demographic data, including, age, sex, height, and weight. Clinical data to be collected from patients' medical records include history of diabetes, type of glucose control/ treatment, diet or medical management, and serum glucose value obtained during routine preoperative visit. In addition, clinical data will include history of renal impairment and immunosuppression. The next data collection point is 10 minutes postincision to catch the body's immune response, repeating a bedside capillary glucometer test. Bedside capillary glucometer testing will continue every hour until surgery completion (surgery is considered completed when the surgical dressing is applied). These times were chosen to ensure an intraoperative draw on short orthopedic procedures < 1 1/2 hours. These time intervals are based on standard ICU glucose monitoring orders due to the stress of hyperglycemia.

Results: To be determined
Conclusions: To be determined

REFERENCES

Mraovic, B., Minarcik, B. A., Hipszer, B. R., Grunwald, Z., & Joseph, J. I. (2006). Glucose management in orthopedic surgery patients. *Anesthesiology, 105,* A381.

Streeter, N. B., & Haley, J. A. (2006, May/June). Considerations in prevention of surgical site infections following cardiac surgery: When your patient is diabetic. *Cardiovascular Nursing, 21*(3), E14–E20.

Van den Berghe, G., Wilmer, A., Hermans, G., Meersseman, W., Wouters, P. J., & Milants, I. (2006). Intensive insulin therapy in the medical ICU. *New England Journal of Medicine, 5,* 449–461.

CHAPTER 51

Sailing into Research

Amy E. Winecoff

Where do I start? I am the director of employee health and worker's compensation for a 105-bed hospital in a growing town in rural North Carolina. Nursing is not my first degree. I also have a degree in biology with a minor in psychology. All my life, I have loved numbers and creating change for the good. I belong to the Association of American Occupational Health Nurses, and I actually proofread continuing education and research articles for my association's journal. My problem was getting the backbone to make it happen for myself. My biggest fear was of rejection or even being laughed at for thinking that what I had done equaled research. I totally lacked confidence, but the research council at Lake Norman Regional Medical Center (LNRMC) changed that. A professor in the School of Nursing at the University of North Carolina at Charlotte gave me not only a backbone but also a master's-prepared nursing student to help me on my quest.

When I began keeping track of the Occupational Safety & Health Administration (OSHA) log and doing employee health and worker's compensation, the one trend that kept popping up was minor back injuries. I tried to see if LNRMC had a class for refreshing the employees on proper lifting, and there was not one. At about this time, LNRMC hired a new director for the Rehabilitation Department. I approached him, and we discussed the injury rate and decided that we needed to try and make a change. We created the back class. All new employees go through this during orientation and repeat it if injured on the job. The class is standardized for orientation, but for injuries, it is related to how the employee became injured. The employees must report all back injuries to Employee Health. Employee Health calls or e-mails Rehab with the employee's name. It is the employee's responsibility to call and make the appointment with Rehab to take the class. It is a one-on-one class. The employee describes and shows the physical therapist how the injury occurred, and the therapist teaches the employee how to avoid harming himself or herself if he or she is in that situation again. The therapist also gives the employee exercises to do at home to strengthen the injured area.

The other change made was to channel all back injuries through the same physician, who is also my medical director. She and I met and mapped out a treatment plan for all back sprains and strains. If injuries are more severe, medical treatment overrides the class until the employee is ready for physical therapy. This also bumped the employee from the study. I looked at the numbers. I had no game plan in 2001, so the numbers were not bad, but we wanted to know if we had in fact made a difference. This is where the professor of the school of nursing was so gracious in giving me a master's-prepared nursing student to help me write what I had done and to help with all the statistics, institutional review board procedures, and so on. The student helped me to put all the data together. Our numbers in 2001 were an average of 5.6 lost work days per back injury, and 8.8 days of light duty. The numbers at the end of 2006—at the end of our study and after the start of the back class—were an average of 1.113 lost work days and 3.92 light duty days. The most amazing discovery was that our average cost of a back injury decreased, from $2,266.48 to—are you ready for this—$364.81. The best part was that we decided to submit what we wrote to *Nursing Economic$*, which accepted our article on the first submission.

I felt like I had climbed Mount Everest! My game plan worked, and it continues to prove itself. I now realize that research does not have to be in a large teaching facility, and it does not have to be direct patient care. My research helped indirectly with patient care by keeping my staff healthier and better able to care at the bedside. I actually began to believe in myself. I can't wait to decide what my next trend to change will be and show how research can create change for the better.

My advice to anyone who wants to do research is to just do it. Look at trends. Are they good, or could they be improved? Make the change and document the change, for better or for worse. Plenty of help is available from local universities' nursing or statistics departments. Read articles on what it is you want to change; see if it has been done before to determine if you can replicate it in your setting. Remember that nothing ventured is nothing gained!

Cost and Clinical Outcomes of a Back Injury Clinic

Amy E. Winecoff, BSN, RN, COHN-S

Purpose: The researchers asked if the use of a back injury class/clinic made a difference in employee and organizational outcomes after a work-related back injury.

Design: The study was built on a feasible evidence-based protocol for a small hospital. The study focused primarily on the response and intervention after a lower back injury occurred. The researchers compared data from before the initiation of the back clinic with data collected after the initiation of the back clinic. The time span was January 2001 to December 2006.

Methods: Prior to the establishment of the back clinic, an injured employee would go to the hospital's emergency department and then follow up with whomever he or she chose to see, or not be seen at all. Once the back injury clinic was established, employees with a lower back injury reported to Employee Health. Employee Health sent the employee's name to Rehab, and an appointment was made with the medical director of Employee Health. The medical director followed the protocol set in place and prescribed the back class and physical therapy if needed. If warranted, the employee was sent to a specialist. To be included in the study, the employee had to have a lower back injury that occurred on the job and that was related in some way to lifting. The University of North Carolina at Charlotte is our research partner, and its institutional review board approved the research study. All data were obtained from the Occupational Safety & Health Administration (OSHA) logs from each year, and the paid costs were obtained from the third-party carrier. Days lost and light duty days, in which another employee replaced the injured employee, doubled the dollar amount of salary for the day lost. All comparisons were conducted using a two-tailed t test. The significance level was adjusted for multiple comparisons using the Bonferroni adjustment. Criterion for statistical significance was $p < 0.0228$, with the assumption that variances were equal.

Results: Prior to the establishment of the back clinic, the average lost time was 5.6 days per back injury, and light duty was 8.8 days per back injury. The average costs of the back injuries were $2,266.48. After the establishment of the back clinic, the average days lost dropped to 1.13 days per back injury, and light duty dropped to 3.92 days. The biggest change was the cost per injury; the cost of a back injury after the implementation of the clinic dropped to $364.81.

Conclusions: At Lake Norman Regional Medical Center, the use of a back clinic led to the following positive economic outcomes: reduced costs, fewer lost days, and a quicker return to full duty from light duty. The back clinic also provided the following clinical outcomes: increase in employee back strength, increase in employee knowledge, and decrease in employee reinjury. As shown in previous studies, the study found that a well-structured back injury clinic is an integral part of a comprehensive effort to control worker's compensation claims related to duration and cost.

CHAPTER 52

You've Got Mail

Paula Lomas

I was fortunate to find my niche in nursing early in my career. I found myself in 1988 as a nurse coordinator of a cystic fibrosis (CF) center. By 1990, I was also involved in clinical trials for this unique patient population. As a research coordinator, I was encouraged by the fact that I could be part of a team of pathfinders in developing treatments for this worthy group of individuals: They were born with a chronic genetic progressive disease that would surely bring them an early death.

I was satisfied for a while to collect data for someone else, but as time went on, I saw the opportunity to conduct my own nursing research. I was enrolled in a management theory class and was intrigued by the various motivational theories presented. What motivated the nurse coordinator to continue working with this patient population? The stress related to caring for chronic terminal patients did not seem to affect the turnover rate of this nursing group. I would see the same faces at our annual CF meetings. I myself was in this profession for many years. In light of the present nursing shortage, I theorized that the turnover rate for this nursing subgroup was very low. My professor encouraged me to send out a survey to measure the turnover rate. My survey was sent out via e-mail to nurse coordinators of accredited CF centers with the help of my nurse contact at the Cystic Fibrosis Foundation (CFF). Within minutes of my survey being distributed, I had 30 responses! How exciting it was to see the pop-up icon on my computer continually saying, "You've got mail." The response by my colleagues was overwhelming. Ultimately, I received responses from over 100 CF nurse coordinators.

This awesome response led me to incorporate e-mail surveys into my next nursing research venture. The camaraderie of my colleagues was put to the test. I knew that my peers would be responsive, and they did not disappoint me. This wonderful group of nurses proved to be supportive and receptive to my call for help, yet again. How reassuring it is to know that there is a group of nurses who support, encourage, and assist me in my endeavor to embrace nursing research.

It was my experience that there was a small number of patients with cystic fibrosis who had given birth to or fathered a child with this terminal illness. This has not been documented in the literature. I asked my colleagues once again to answer a survey. I mailed surveys addressed to nurse coordinators. The response rate was 34% using this method. I then again went to my nurse contact at the CFF and asked her to send out an e-mail of this survey to the same CF centers to which I had mailed surveys. Again, this method proved to be extremely effective. My response rate increased to 83% using this technology. For a second time, I watched my e-mail inbox fill with responses. I was so excited; it was like getting responses to a party!

When reviewing abstracts for the annual North American Cystic Fibrosis conference, I was disappointed that there was a small number of nursing abstract submissions. Some nurses had performed quality improvement projects and submitted abstracts under that category. However, as often occurs, nurses are putting the needs of others before themselves. We need to question what we are doing, why we are doing it, and if we are doing it in the best way. The nurse coordinators are busy with other duties; nursing research goes on the back burner as something they would like to do—someday. Perhaps I will need to become a champion for this group and encourage them to delve into the exciting and rewarding world of nursing research.

I encourage novice nursing researchers to network with other nurses and contacts they have in the communities they serve. For me, e-mail seemed to be a very effective method to gain responses from the nursing group with whom I work. Encourage other nurses to "invite people to your party." Ask them to respond to your invitation to research. You will be very excited to view the response you will receive.

The Estimated Incidence of Patients with Cystic Fibrosis (CF) Having a CF-Affected Child: A Survey of CF Centers Throughout the United States

Paula Lomas, BSN, RN, CCRP

Purpose: The purpose of this study is to identify the number of CF adults who have children affected with CF in the United States.

Background: The Adult CF Center at Morristown Memorial Hospital follows 4 (6%) patients with CF who have children also diagnosed with this disease. Each parent was diagnosed after his or her child. The CF patient data registry cannot identify the patients with CF who have CF children. As the average age of survival has increased, so has the likelihood of CF patients having CF offspring.

Method: A six-question survey was sent to CF care centers via standard mail or facsimile based on information from the CF Center Directory. A total of 144 questionnaires addressed to the center nurse coordinator were sent. One month after the last survey was sent, an e-mail reminder was distributed by the Cystic Fibrosis Foundation (CFF).

Results: Prior to an e-mail reminder, 50 (34%) responses were returned. After the e-mail reminder, an additional 69 questionnaires were returned, for a total of 119 responses, an 83% response rate. The number of parents with CF having children with CF numbered 66. Of those, 27 (41%) were diagnosed before pregnancy, and 39 (59%) were diagnosed after their children. The majority of those diagnosed after their children were diagnosed as a result of their child's diagnosis (86%). Only 3 (8%) were diagnosed as a result of prenatal testing.

Conclusion: Based on the number of adults with CF in the United States (10,039), the incidence of CF adults having CF children is < 1%. This incidence may increase as age of survival increases. The CFF may choose to link parent and child. Potential physical and psychosocial impacts can then be tracked. Centers were more likely to respond to e-mailed surveys. Nursing researchers should consider this method when surveying nurses.

CHAPTER 53

Getting Started in Research— You Can Do It with a Little Nudge

Barb Bungard

My initial direct involvement with nursing research happened by accident, thanks to a vendor. My role at the time was as a nurse educator for the pediatric intensive care unit (PICU), and we were addressing the issue of special care beds and skin breakdown. There was, and unfortunately still is, limited research available regarding skin breakdown in the pediatric population and the use of an appropriate pediatric assessment tool. Pediatric patients traditionally do not have a large number of skin integrity issues, though this should not be an excuse for not doing a comprehensive assessment.

The sales representative working with our hospital was aware of our interest in special care beds and skin breakdown, and she contacted me. The sales rep asked me if our institution was interested in being part of a multicenter study whose purpose was to explore the prevalence of skin breakdown in the pediatric population and validate a specific assessment tool for pediatrics.

Having never been directly involved with research, this study interested me. The study protocol was already developed, samples of the proposal were available to take to the institutional review board (IRB), and, most important, it was very time limited—a 1-day observation. In addition, the vendor would assist us in the data collection and forward our data to the coordinating institution. Resources needed on our end were limited.

Prior to this study research was not something I read or understood, nor was it a process with which I had the time to be actively involved. I thought nurses provided bedside care and that research was conducted by those in academia. I had an interest in research, but I did not think I had the skills or ability to lead a study at our hospital.

Our pediatric institution has limited resources available to support research efforts, especially in nursing. We do not have dedicated data entry staff. We do have an individual from the nursing department on the IRB committee who has a strong research background and who eagerly serves as a mentor, especially for those just getting started in research.

I approached this person and asked her if she thought this research project was feasible, if she would help me, and what I needed to do to make it work. She said, "We can do it, it is a great opportunity, and I would love to help you." So, I called the vendor back and said to count us in!

One of the driving forces for our interest was our institution's lack of coordinated skin assessment practices. Several of the specific areas within the hospital conducted their own skin assessments, and the practices for treatment were not standardized. We do not have skin/wound integrity specialists. Our nursing staff often struggle to address skin integrity issues, having questions such as whom to contact and what works best. The hope was that with results from the study, we would be able to establish standardized skin care practices for our patients.

A meeting was held with the vendor staff and our nursing staff at Children's. Because we did not have wound specialists, we identified advanced practice nurses who would examine and stage wounds found on the study day. The core group of nursing staff was educated on the Modified Braden Q tool prior to the study. This tool is used as a predictor of pressure ulcer risk in pediatric patients. The tool uses a scoring matrix to examine mobility, sensory perception, and tissue perfusion/oxygenation in our patients. The study was approved by our IRB and is still active. Submitting the proposal to the IRB was a learning experience. All the members of the research committee were much more experienced than I was with the nursing research process, but I knew that I was being an advocate for the patients we care for and that this study was important.

Gaining consent prior to the study was our first challenge. Because of our short length of stay, it was decided we would seek consent the night before the study. This became a challenge, though, because several parents were not at the bedside to give consent for the study. Some of the patients were able to give assent because of their age, but not consent. We did get consent for approximately 75% of the patients admitted to the hospital on the study day. The study was completed, and the results generated no surprises. The results did support our frustration with an uncoordinated approach to this topic. Specific populations are at a higher risk and prevalence for skin breakdown and need our expertise.

So, how did I feel after the study? I was excited, but frustrated. The excitement came from having all the pieces fall together and knowing that we were successful. The study also was published. Energy radiated from nurses who had never completed bedside research before. Actual practice did change in our neonatal intensive care unit (NICU) regarding heel sticks from blood draws. The PICU has adopted the Modified Braden Q as a skin assessment tool for all patients. In addition, through collaboration with the trauma services, skin breakdown protocols are being used based on the Modified Braden Q scores. However, there is frustration because of the realization of inadequate resources at our institution to move other components of the study forward. We do not have dedicated research staff within most of the clinical areas. After three years, we still do not have a standardized approach to assessment of skin breakdown even though we have participated in follow-up studies for over three years. Through all the follow-up studies, we have not seen definite trends of at-risk pediatric patients, except for the critical care areas. As a result, the urgency to change practice does not exist, but it will come.

My advice for future researchers is, "Go for it!" Networking is key for novice researchers to get their feet wet. Start small by collecting data; suggest an idea that needs to be looked at within your practice. Listen, read, and talk with your peers. Nothing is impossible. Patience and persistence are necessary at times. Use the resources around you. Foundation money is not just for the doctors. If you don't ask, you will never know what is available. Find a mentor or ally to guide you along the way.

Acknowledgment: I would like to thank and acknowledge the support I received from my mentor, Dr. Aris Eliades, throughout this project. Her patience, guidance, and expertise have been essential as I started this process and continue to gain experience in nursing research.

Assessing Prevalence of Pressure Ulcer and Skin Breakdown in a Children's Hospital

Barb Bungard, BSN, RN, CCRN

Purpose: Document the prevalence of skin breakdown and pressure ulcers in hospitalized children.

Design: A descriptive study that includes existing documentation in the medical record and physical assessments of hospitalized children under the age of 18 years.

Methods: Prevalence of pressure ulcers and skin breakdown was measured on a predetermined day and period of time in the nine participating children's hospitals. For each patient, a physical skin assessment was performed, and all found that pressure ulcers were staged according to the National Pressure Ulcer Advisory Panel staging system. Demographics and potential risk factors were obtained from documentation within the medical record. The Neonatal/Infant Braden Q Risk Assessment was used to score infants younger than 1 year, and the Braden Q Risk Assessment was used for children older than 1 year. Data collection forms were completed and entered into the FAST data collection software. The data were analyzed at a central site at the end of the day.

Results: A total of 1,064 children (75 children at Akron Children's Hospital) were surveyed from the nine hospitals, with a pressure ulcer prevalence of 4%, and other skin breakdown prevalence of 14.8%. The percentages at Akron Children's Hospital were similar for pressure ulcers (6.7%), though significantly higher for skin breakdown (40%). The increase in skin breakdown was identified to be in the neonatal population from blood draws in the heels.

Facility-acquired skin breakdown was 2.7% in the nine hospitals and at Akron. The three most common types of skin breakdown were excoriation/diaper dermatitis, skin tear, and IV extravasation. Predominant locations for skin breakdown were seat area, 35% (Akron 17%); foot area, 20% (Akron 35%); and upper extremities, 18% (Akron 4%).

Conclusions: The prevalence of pressure ulcers was low in the pediatric population studied, but actual skin breakdown was higher. Future pediatric specific studies are needed to evaluate prevention and treatment options, including periodic review for benchmarking purposes.

CHAPTER 54

Reflection of a Nursing Research Journey: From Conception to Completion

Wendy Ploegstra

Prior to embarking on my recent research journey, I was intrigued by the nursing research process and had great respect for the use of research findings in my nursing practice. It was in my graduate school research course that I discovered this process to be fascinating, and I actually enjoyed it. I did have fears that being involved in research meant that I would not be able to spend as much time in clinical practice. It seemed to me that you could choose to be a good clinician and use evidence-based practice (EBP), or you could be a nurse researcher and create EBP. I did not think it was possible to do both, so I decided that I was more interested in patient care and that patient care was where my focus would be. When I decided to get my master's, I chose a school with a reputation of having more strength in developing nurse practitioners (NPs) with "clinical practice" as opposed to "research," which other competing schools prided themselves upon. I hoped that at some point in my career, I would have the opportunity to help out with a research study and learn more about conducting real research.

The problem that led me to my current research interest occurred early in my nursing career. As a new BSN grad, I chose to work in the pediatric intensive care unit (PICU) because I enjoyed children, and the intensity of the ICU setting appealed to me. Beginning my career in such an intensity-driven environment was a difficult transition, and many days I wondered if I would last a year, or even six months. I committed myself to give at least a year and would not allow myself to give up. Every day that I left the PICU, I was exhausted physically, mentally, and emotionally. One of the biggest stressors that I experienced was related to patient loss in the PICU. Though I always felt truly privileged to comfort and guide a family through the very difficult time of losing a child, I often felt that the support system was not adequate.

I decided to seek out support from our chaplain at the time, because I heard she was concerned about addressing the psychosocial needs of nurses in the unit. We discussed the need for greater emotional support of nurses in the PICU setting and brainstormed ideas to meet this deficiency. Unfortunately, after discussing the possibility of applying for a grant to help fund our ideas, that chaplain left, and it seemed that my ideas fell to the wayside. I wasn't sure how to proceed and felt overwhelmed by continuing the process on my own, so about a year or so went by with nothing done. During this interim period, we had short-term chaplains come and go, which didn't allow our ideas to get off the ground. After some time, the children's hospital got a new full-time chaplain, and after a short period, we began to have discussions regarding the psychosocial needs of the nurses. He had recognized a severe lack of support for the nursing staff in terms of grief and bereavement. At the same time, I was in the process of deciding on a topic for my master's capstone project, and the ideas collided. Ultimately, we decided that if we were to implement a program for nursing support, we needed to begin by adequately assessing the nurses' needs. This is where the research idea began!

I definitely feel empowered. The journey thus far has been very challenging and demanding, but each day I seem to make a little progress and try to focus on the end result. My hope is that I will ultimately be able to give something back to improve our profession of nursing. I can better appreciate the rigor and intensity of conducting research after this experience, and I am more appreciative of the research that others have done to allow me to apply these EBP strategies in my own practice.

Think big and have a vision. Then seek out a mentor who will guide you along the way and offer continual encouragement that what you are doing will eventually pay off. I feel extremely blessed to have had such an incredible mentor to guide me in the process and break it down into pieces that I could digest. If you look at it as one giant piece to swallow, you will be too overwhelmed to even begin, so you must break it down into bite-sized pieces. This is no doubt hard work, and you need support. You need someone to help you through the difficult parts and help you recognize the small achievements that you will make along the way. There are many achievements along the research journey besides the final project. Every step along the way, you will learn and grow. Don't expect to do it all by yourself; engage team members and, if possible, seek out interdisciplinary team members to impact organization-wide initiatives. Other disciplines can offer insights that you may not have picked up on by yourself. Diversify the body so that the project is more complete and will speak to a greater variety of readers.

I will conclude with the top 10 things I learned along my research journey:

10. Learn about the IRB process at your institution and at your university if your study is also a school project.
 9. Share your project with others to gain buy-in from the get-go.

8. There will be countless revisions! Don't take it personally.
7. Establish a reasonable timeline and be prepared for setbacks.
6. Break it up into small, manageable chunks.
5. A comprehensive literature review is imperative to begin and to finish well.
4. Be persistent.
3. Choose a topic that you are passionate about; you will need that passion to get you through the tough parts.
2. Enlist a multidisciplinary team to be involved in the project.
1. Establish a mentor.

Acknowledgment: The author would like to acknowledge the expertise of nurse researcher Dr. Janice Phillips for the guidance, patience, and expertise she provided to me as a novice researcher.

Determinants of Burnout in PICU Nurses

Wendy Ploegstra, MSN, RN, CCRN; Janice Phillips, PhD, RN;
Eric Price, MDiv; and Sarah Hoehn, MD

Background and Significance: Significant stressors, including critical incident stress, are a prevalent risk for burnout in critical care nursing. Yet, there appear to be limited reported interventions that aid in the prevention of burnout among critical care nurses. It is likely that the pediatric intensive care unit (PICU) nurse experiences burnout differently than his or her adult counterparts do, and there is little research to assess the uniqueness of their experiences. Additionally, there is a lack of published interventions to address burnout and prevent the damaging effects of this syndrome.

Purpose: The purpose of this two-phase study was to examine the prevalence of and contributing factors related to burnout in PICU nurses.

Design: A descriptive exploratory design was used to (1) establish the prevalence of burnout among pediatric nurses and (2) identify the determinants of burnout in PICU nurses.

Methods: During Phase I, 68 staff nurses completed the Maslach Burnout Inventory-Human Services Survey (MBI-HSS), which examines the demographic characteristics, occupational experience, perceived job workload, exercise of control, reward and recognition for work done, sense of community, fairness, and match of personal values with institution values. During Phase II, 15 nurses participated in focus group discussions that involved a more detailed discussion of the variables identified in Phase I. Focus group participants also identified strategies for promoting well-being and positive coping among PICU nurses.

Results: The mean frequency rates (with standard deviation) of the entire sample were 21.8 (9.2), 7.6 (4.7), and 34.7 (6.4) for emotional exhaustion, depersonalization, and personal accomplishment, respectively. No significant differences in levels of emotional exhaustion, depersonalization, or personal accomplishment were found using a one-way analysis of variance (ANOVA) comparison in all the demographic variables ($p < 0.05$). Focus groups provided a rich understanding of the specific stressors that may contribute to burnout.

Conclusion: Findings from this study will help to provide a framework for the design and implementation of an evidence-based protocol to promote effective stress management in the PICU nurse.

CHAPTER 55

My Research Surprise

Carol Swartz

I thought our practice was "doing it right" for nebulization treatment of infants and began my journey to encourage the rest of our physician network practices also to "do it right." I began with a literature search and found a big surprise.

When our community hospital began its Magnet journey, I didn't pay much attention to the talk about evidence-based practice and nursing research. I work in a busy pediatric clinic and just didn't have time for more paperwork and other "nonsense." I had always thought of research as being done by a PhD candidate or university professor. Certainly not by me, a nurse for 42 years with absolutely no research experience. In fact, I would sometimes shake my head and muse, *Don't these nursing leaders think we have anything better to do with our time?*

As our hospital's journey toward Magnet recognition progressed, our nursing leaders continued to encourage us to ask research questions. I would hear this mentioned frequently in the nursing committee meetings I attended each month and had to admit to myself that there was a question that was nagging at me: *Is there research to support the benefits of using a mask to administer pediatric nebulizer treatments versus using the "blow-by" method?* In our practice, we have always used masks because one of our nurse practitioners has asthma and insisted on it.

Sometimes I covered in another network office on weekends, and they had no masks because they did only blow-by. We would often have to repeat a treatment because the child kept wheezing. I asked myself, *Does this mean the medication is "blowing by" the patient?*

I became excited as my review of the literature progressed because I discovered in several articles that there was research evidence to support using a mask rather than blow-by to give infants nebulization treatments. I was surprised that the evidence supported having a tight seal between the infant's face and mask rim. Moving a mask just 1 or 2 cm from the face decreases drug efficacy by 59% to 85%, respectively. We were not using tight-fitting masks in our clinic, and I couldn't find them. I became frustrated and concerned that we would never locate the correct equipment. I contacted several resources, including the pediatric pulmonology office affiliated with the university hospital that follows many of our patients. They informed me that they use blow-by for their patients.

One day, I was discussing my literature search results with a pharmaceutical representative. The vendor's literature stated that a tight-fitting mask should be used. The pharmaceutical representative referred me to a study that compared jet nebulizers and gave me the name of the vendor's representative. This equipment provided the greatest efficacy. We were given samples of the masks. Not only could we get masks sized to our patients instead of the "one size fits all" previously used, but also, the nebulizer that came with them provided better efficacy related to nebulization time and amount of drug delivered.

The entire process took much longer than I had anticipated. However, knowing that we were able to improve outcomes for our little patients has been worth it all, and I feel a great sense of satisfaction. I would encourage all nurses to "ask the question" and use the resources available in their particular hospital to get started. I was fortunate because our hospital has a research nurse who was very supportive and a great resource as I began the process.

Acknowledgment: My research surprise never would have happened without the vision of Linda Miller, CNO, for our hospital to travel the Magnet journey. I also want to offer my gratitude for the immense support that I received on my research journey from the providers I work with each day: Dr. Padmaraju and the following FNPs: Jeannette Hadwin, Marjorie Langevin, and Karen Whelan. I especially want to extend my thanks to Fran Anderson, PhD, nurse researcher, who has been a wonderful resource and my constant encourager. Last but not least, my thanks and appreciation to Angela Martz, the Astra Zeneca representative who came to my rescue when I didn't know where else to turn.

Blow-by versus Face Mask for Infant/Pediatric Nebulization Treatments

Carol Swartz, RN

Purpose: The purpose of our pilot study was to answer the question, Is the use of a specific tight-fitting mask effective for delivering nebulization treatments to infants and small children?

Design: Convenience sampling was used to select 8 pediatric patients as subjects who required nebulization treatments.

Methods: Subjects selected were patients who had been receiving nebulizer treatments with the old equipment. Treatments using the new equipment were observed in the clinic by providers, nurses, and parents. The clinical outcome measures of decreased wheezing and improved breath sounds also were measured.

Results: Providers and staff reported better efficacy related to the new masks and finer mist/better absorption of medications, as evidenced by increased respiratory quality post-nebulizer treatments. The new equipment was more convenient to use because treatments could be given while a child was lying on his or her back and sleeping. An unexpected finding was that parents and staff both noted that the new equipment was much quieter, and children tended to be less agitated during treatments.

Conclusions: This pilot study was so successful that it led to a change in practice for delivering nebulization treatments to infants and small children within both hospital and outpatient settings.

(2006)

CHAPTER 56

90 Percent of Life Is Just Showing Up

Cynthia Earley

Research?! It may sound corny, but I became a nurse to help people. I embrace the drama, intensity, and rewards of direct patient care. How satisfying it is to see that my efforts can actually help people regain their strength, their joy, and return home to family and friends. In other cases, it is no less rewarding to be there during the final stages of a patient's life to comfort and care for him or her. That is why I became a nurse, and it is what gets me up in the morning.

Why, then, would I want to do research? Like most, I am fearful when I am out of my comfort zone, and research seemed way out of my comfort zone. As a return-to-practice nurse who had been out of the hospital for decades, I had struggled enough to get back on my feet as a nurse on a postsurgical unit. The whole world of evidence-based practice had passed me by. What little contact I had with actual research, going back to when I was a student nurse volunteering to participate in research studies conducted at the University of Virginia School of Nursing. That was two decades ago!

But like many new ventures in life begin, someone tapped me on the shoulder and asked me if I would get involved. The need was for a nurse who was available to represent the postsurgical unit on our research council. Being fairly new, I wanted to show that I was willing to be a team player, but I was reluctant and unsure about being up to the task.

My foray into the world of research was tenuous at first—ICFs, IRBs, t tests, z scores? What were all these terms? I felt like I was starting at the bottom again. Sitting at the conference table with the interdisciplinary members of the research council, I struggled to absorb the importance of the ongoing research studies, literature reviews, and acronyms that accompanied it all. I was definitely an unlikely participant in this world.

Fortunately, the research council meetings were varied and interesting. I continued to attend for several months when a topic of particular interest to me presented itself: childhood obesity. On the postsurgical unit, I had been observing the devastating consequences of adult patients with diabetes. They were entering the hospital for treatment of various conditions of their disease that were complicated by their weight status. This was a different population from the patients I saw as a nurse 20 years ago. If only I could intervene before their health condition deteriorated. . . . Childhood obesity seemed a vital target for research.

My attention was focused when volunteers were requested from our research council to assist in a childhood obesity study that was just being initiated. The skills needed were the ability to take accurate height and weight measurements and to calculate body mass index. I was there.

The Woody Allen quote, "90% of life is just showing up" is the title of my story. After showing up as a nurse helper, I became much more deeply involved in this research study. Because I had completed the National Institute of Health module on human subject protection, I was able to assist with the completion of informed consents for many of the 185 participants. Although I was not initially involved in developing the protocol of this study, we submitted a request to the institutional review board (IRB) to add my name as a subinvestigator. This became the vehicle for a wealth of experience. Assisting in the 6-month implementation of this study, I saw firsthand the challenges of nursing research: painstaking data collection, adherence to protocol, and measures that needed to be taken to comply with the regard for human subject protection. Then came the data input. This was another level of challenge, because I had never even worked with Excel spreadsheets before. More tasks prevailed for me to accomplish: quality assurance of the data, verification of statistical analysis, writing for journal publication, and editing, writing, and rewriting. Eventually, publication in the December 2007 issue of the *Journal of School Nursing* was the reward. Shortly thereafter, the local newspaper wrote about childhood obesity and cited our study and its findings.

I attribute my satisfying experience with research to three key factors: mentoring, teamwork, and continuing education. If I was offering advice to other nurses, I would encourage them to seek out opportunities such as these.

Mentoring. The most crucial element of mentoring was available through our director of nursing research who is also the chair of the research council. She guides nursing research from the conceptual stages through implementation and publication. Successful mentoring includes preparing a person with skills and giving him or her the opportunity to practice those skills with guidance and feedback. As an example, after receiving training in human subject protection, I was given the opportunity to observe the informed consent process. That quickly moved to responsibilities for obtaining informed consent and assent in two different research studies. After more experience, I was asked to prepare a review of the informed consent process for our research council. Knowing the value of repetition, my mentor then worked with me to refine the content and present again for a wider audience at a clinical research course offered by our hospital. Using the novice-to-expert model, mentoring was the vehicle that enabled me to develop competence in this area.

Teamwork. The opportunity to be a member of the research council has provided opportunities to hear ideas for research studies and to see those ideas shaped by discussion and constructive criticism. Opportunities to work with others on their research studies have given me a wealth of exposure to different protocols, case review forms, and various statistical tests.

Continuing education. As I was moving along this path of research, I was also discovering the wealth of opportunities for continuing education, even without pursuing an advanced degree. I took advantage of many in-services, conferences, and poster presentations, which filled in my knowledge gaps. Librarians taught me how to write with the American Psychological Association writing style and how to use the RefWorks system. Nurses spoke on writing for publication, and I completed a 2-day clinical research course and an Inova Research Day. Not only was the content valuable, but also the opportunity to intersect with other nurses who were conducting research was an education in itself.

As things progressed, I realized that my fears had been much ado about nothing. My love for patient care was only being enriched as I was plunged into nursing research. What I was learning in research made me sharper on the floor. Likewise, my daily patient contact kept my feet anchored in the real world as I engaged in research. Much like the paradigm of the soldier/scholar, I was finding that the paradigm of the nurse/researcher was incredibly rewarding and a dynamite combination.

A Prospective Study Comparing Obesity-Related Outcomes Between Kids Living Fit™ and Elementary School Contrast Students

Karen Gabel Speroni, PhD, RN; Cynthia Earley, BSN, RN; and Martin Atherton, DrPH

Purpose: The Centers for Disease Control and Prevention (CDC) reported that from 1999–2000 through 2003–2004, the prevalence of overweight status among children ages 2–19 years increased from 14.0% to 18.2% among males and from 13.8% to 16.0% among females (Ogden et al., 2006). Lacking in recent research literature is the effect that schools might have in both preventing overweight status among normal-weight children and reversing unhealthy body mass index (BMI) status among overweight children. To facilitate improved lifestyle choices for children with respect to activities chosen and foods consumed, community hospital nurses, over a series of three studies, designed an intervention, Kids Living Fit™[1] (KLF), and tested whether it could effect change in participants' BMI for age and gender when implemented as an after-school program. The KLF intervention included exercise and dietary education components, as well as interventions by nurses.

The objective of this study was to provide a volunteer after-school-based program that enhances the health and physical education curriculum for elementary school-age children in order to decrease overweight and maintain healthy weights. This would be accomplished through teaching healthy lifestyle choices of best choice foods and demonstration and teaching of active behaviors. The study hypothesis is that the KLF intervention group will significantly decrease their average BMI percentile, adjusted for age (months) and gender,

---

[1]*Kids Living Fit™ is an exercise program designed and offered by Good Sports Fitness, LLC, Leesburg, Virginia.*

as compared with the contrast group, and maintain healthy weights in the KLF group as compared with the contrast group.

Design: This was a prospective, quasi-experimental design study comparing an exercise and dietary education after-school program intervention (KLF) with a contrast group receiving no intervention. The IRB approved the study. Informed consent was obtained. This study was conducted in four public schools located in the community served by the hospital.

Methods: All participants were followed through Week 24. For both groups, measures for height, weight, and waist circumference were recoded at baseline, Week 12, and Week 24, and activity and food choice satisfaction questionnaires were completed by the participants. Additional intervention exercise and dietary education were provided for the KLF group. The KLF exercise component was taught by a physical fitness trainer for one hour weekly for 12 consecutive weeks at elementary schools in Loudoun County. The program focused on physical fitness (e.g., aerobic dance, basic muscle groups, light strength training, stretching, balancing techniques, and student heart rate monitoring associated with exercise), yoga, and relaxation techniques (e.g., meditation, breathing). During four of the 12 weeks (i.e., Weeks 1, 4, 8, and 12), the KLF program was held for 30 minutes. For the additional 30 minutes, the registered dietitians presented balanced nutrition lectures at these four time points. Parents were encouraged to attend, and parental attendance was measured.

Participants completed food and activity diaries and wore pedometers at various time points throughout the study.

Results: There were 185 participants (KLF group = 80; contrast group = 105) who were followed to Week 24. A higher percentage of females were enrolled in the KLF group than the contrast group (57% vs. 44%, $p < 0.05$). The majority of students enrolled in the KLF group were in Grade 4 (29%), whereas the majority (33%) were in Grade 2 in the contrast group.

In pairwise comparisons, the KLF group realized a significant decrease as compared with the contrast group in BMI percentile between baseline and follow-up (–2.3%). The KLF group demonstrated a smaller increase in waist circumference than the contrast group.

Conclusions: The KLF program provides methodologies for an exercise and dietary education after-school-based program to teach best lifestyle choices to elementary school-age children and reduce BMI.

The fact that nearly half of the KLF group who were overweight or at risk of becoming overweight perceived their body image as "just right" supports the need for educating children and their parents on BMI results and associated ramifications of being overweight.

Nurses can encourage children to make best lifestyle choices with respect to foods consumed and activities chosen to increase the potential for a lifetime of normal weight.

REFERENCES

Ogden, C. L., Carroll, M. D., Curtin, L. R., McDowell, M. A., Tabak, C.J., & Flegal, K. M. (2006). Prevalence of overweight and obesity in the United States, 1999–2004. *Journal of the American Medical Association, 295*(13), 1549–1555.

CHAPTER 57

Research and Me, You Must Be Kidding

Jane H. Hartman

My first negative feelings about research began with my first class in graduate school, statistics—4 hours a night, 2 nights a week for 5 weeks. Who thinks up this stuff? Needless to say, it was grueling, and the only thing that saved me was the take-home tests. The second reason I knew I'd never do research was my graduate research class. We had to review an article once a week and decipher the statistics in the article—boring, dry, and non-motivating to someone with two teenage boys, a husband, and a dog at home, all wanting a piece of me.

The problem that led to my involvement in research was a new job as a sedation nurse in pediatric radiology in a prestigious hospital in a large urban city. The problem was that we had no educational materials, no plan, and no child life staff to help these children with anxiety and stress related to the test procedure. Educational issues involved inserting catheters for intravenous (IV) medications and contrast and having a child lie perfectly still in a large, loud magnetic resonance (MR) scanning machine. I wanted to communicate preparatory information and have everyone else improve their communication to children as well.

My research started as a result of an assignment during my last semester in graduate school. I never planned on implementing this project until I met our director of nursing research at the Cleveland Clinic. She was instrumental in giving me all the assistance that a novice needs to move forward in research. I am currently still conducting the study, but I feel really good about what I have accomplished to date. It has not been a "walk in the park," but I have learned a tremendous lesson and will be better prepared for my next project.

To overcome the fear of research, I would give this advice: If you're passionate about a certain patient population and you want to have an impact on their outcomes, research is the way to go. Prove your point with comparisons and outcomes, and things will change. Research gives you a forum to change things instead of complaining that things never change. They can and will change with evidence-based outcomes.

Decreasing Stress and Anxiety for School-Age Children Undergoing Magnetic Resonance Imaging Using a Photo-Diary

Jane H. Hartman, MSN, RN, CPNP

A randomized controlled study will be conducted. Subjects are school-age children undergoing magnetic resonance imaging (MRI) in the neuroradiology MRI area, and parents of children who participate. All subjects provide written informed consent. Inclusion criteria are: Children must be 7–12 years of age, be able to read English, and have the intellectual ability to comprehend the photo-diary and pre- and postsurvey. Children who had prior MRIs before 5 years of age can be included. A child can participate even if his or her parent chooses not to. Children complete two surveys before and after usual care or the intervention that assess anxiety and stress, and demographic data. Parents complete one survey about perceived anxiety of their child at two points. Data have been collected on 30 children and 29 parents. Data analysis is still in process.

CHAPTER 58

Sliding into Research

Irene Huntzinger

I earned a nursing diploma from Good Samaritan School of Nursing in Dayton, Ohio, in 1971 and an associate's degree in science from Edison State College in Piqua, Ohio, in 1982. Neither of these programs incorporated research. As a longtime member of the Association of periOperative Registered Nurses (AORN) Dayton chapter, I did receive some exposure to nursing research. Our AORN chapter research committee, which I joined, performed literature searches and small research studies. The research studies I was aware of took place in the larger hospitals, so my involvement was minimal. I also eagerly joined the newly created research committee at Piqua Memorial Hospital (now Upper Valley Medical Center [UVMC]) in the mid-1980s. As a small hospital, initially our research activity was limited and mostly involved literature searches and then replication studies. Research fascinated me! What a way to discover if something actually worked! We read research books and sometimes I even understood what I was reading. It must be quite obvious that I am a total research novice. I became involved in the research committee at UVMC because it was open to staff nurses, and I so enjoyed learning about research.

One day while in post-anesthesia care unit (PACU), after helping to transport a patient and giving report to the nurse, I was asked by the supervisor and the PACU nurses if we could start using lidocaine jelly as the lubricant for inserting the Foley catheter for abdominal hysterectomy patients. The nurses explained how uncomfortable the patients were post-op, complaining about the Foley. Wait a minute! Just start using lidocaine jelly without knowing if it would work any better? Was this reasonable? Was this smart? What if I conducted a research study? This was the beginning of a long and tedious journey. I really had no idea what I was getting into. Our research committee chair was, and is, my salvation. Her support, along with the whole research team, was essential. I also received much support from my supervisors and coworkers. I did not realize how much work it would be, how much help I would need, or how long it would take. The study took a long time partly because of our limited patient population, but also because I am such a novice and needed help.

The research study is completed! What a feeling of accomplishment! It was well worth the hard work and time involved. All our surgical patients having a

Foley catheter now receive 2% Xylocaine jelly as the catheter lubricant if no allergy is noted. The results showed an improvement in our patients' post-op comfort. I learned more by doing than just reading. I have had new opportunities, I have received recognition for my efforts, and I have inspired other staff nurses to consider doing research.

My advice to other nurses is to be very organized. Have a place you can work from, and keep your data. A computer is very helpful. Enlist the help of your colleagues. I am sure they will be there for you. Join your research committee if you haven't already. The feeling of satisfaction of accomplishing your mission and helping your patients is awesome. If your study doesn't come out as you hoped, it's okay. Research can also show what does not work, which is also very important. Listen to your colleagues. Listen to yourself. What do you think could be improved? What is not working? Grab your idea and do a literature search, and then continue with your research if warranted. You, too, can do it!

Acknowledgment: The author would like to thank Kay Rickey, the UVMC Surgical Services staff, Janet Mullins, Peg Cizadlo, and the UVMC research team for their continued support, encouragement, and assistance. I am blessed by my colleagues' friendship and willingness to help me with my first research project.

Comparison of Immediate Postoperative Complaints of Foley Catheter Discomfort Between Foleys Inserted Using Sterile Lubricant and Sterile 2% Xylocaine Jelly

Irene Huntzinger, RN, CNOR

Purpose: The purpose of the study was to evaluate the effectiveness of 2% Xylocaine jelly use during Foley placement to reduce the immediate post-op discomfort of abdominal hysterectomy patients. Post-anesthesia care unit (PACU) staff reported frequent complaints of needing to void and the general Foley discomfort in abdominal hysterectomy patients. At Upper Valley Medical Center (UVMC), our standard has been to use sterile lubricating jelly (Surgilube) to insert Foley catheters in the operating suite. Other organizations reported using 2% Xylocaine jelly, but no available research was found that supported the reduction in discomfort following the insertion of a Foley catheter using Xylocaine jelly. There is supporting literature on the use of 2% Xylocaine jelly for short-term local anesthesia/analgesia in other applications.

The study was designed to add to the body of evidence-based practice. Review of the literature revealed limited research in this area. The relevance to patient care is to increase patient comfort by reducing the discomfort and sense of urgency associated with a Foley catheter.

Design: The population/sample was 67 abdominal hysterectomy patients who were randomly assigned either to a control group receiving sterile lubricating jelly ($n = 33$) or to a group receiving the 2% Xylocaine jelly ($n = 34$) with catheter insertion. Written consent from the GYN surgeons was obtained prior to the start of the research study.

Method: The setting started in preadmission testing, when the nurse informed patients that they may be part of a research study and received their consent. In operating room (OR), the patients were given the Xylocaine jelly or

Surgilube during insertion of the Foley. The researcher prior to surgery randomly determined which lubricant was used, and the record was kept confidential. The OR nurse began to fill out the data collection tool, and the PACU nurses finished collecting the data. The tool did not indicate which lubricant the patient received, so the PACU nurse was not influenced.

The data collection tool included the date, medical record number, product number, length of surgery, and the OR nurse's initials. The tool continued to PACU, where nurses checked for: c/o needing to void, c/o other catheter complaints, the time the complaints started, whenever the patient was comfortable, if the catheter was secured, and their initials. The data were reported as an aggregate. Janet Mullins, UVMC statistician, assisted in tool design and data analysis. The only potential hazard identified would be a Xylocaine allergy, in which case it would not be used.

Results: A total 67 patients were included in the study; 34 received the 2% Xylocaine jelly, and 33 received Surgilube.

Table 58-1   Catheter Lubricant Results

	Cath with 2% Xylocaine (34)		Cath with Surgilube (33)		Overall 67	
1. Complaint of need to void						
Yes	21%	(7)	45%	(15)	33%	(22)
No	79%	(27)	55%	(18)	67%	(45)
2. Complaint related to catheter						
Yes	24%	(8)	45%	(15)	34%	(23)
No	76%	(26)	55%	(18)	66%	(44)

Chi-square for Item 1 was calculated at 90% and Item 2 at 75%. There was no statistically significant difference based on lubricant type in this study.

Conclusion: Although the chi-square indicated no statistical significance, it was determined that the use of 2% Xylocaine jelly would be implemented for all surgery cases requiring a Foley for the following reasons:

1. Among patients who stayed 206 minutes or more in the PACU (8), only 1 (12.5%) was a patient who had received 2% Xylocaine jelly, whereas 7 (87.5%) patients were from the Surgilube group. With additional costs associated with increased lengths of stay with those receiving Surgilube, it was estimated that approximately $5,213 (in PACU room costs only)

was saved in the 2% Xylocaine group. The cost of using 2% Xylocaine for these 8 patients would be about $26. Although other factors related to increased length of stay were not assessed in this study, surgical services felt that the minimal cost of using 2% Xylocaine jelly was worth the potential savings. If all 67 patients had received 2% Xylocaine, the cost would have been $1,082 (estimated), still showing a savings within the confines of the study.

2. Patient satisfaction—Although patient satisfaction was not measured (no specific comments were made on patient satisfaction surveys), it is assumed that patients prefer to be as comfortable as possible and would not object to an item of minimal cost if it ensured that comfort.

3. Nursing satisfaction—Instituting the 2% Xylocaine as a standard use for OR insertion of Foley catheters was easily implemented. Nurses feel that they are doing more for patient care and comfort and appreciate being heard.

The study should be repeated with a larger sample of patients. Investigating additional factors that may increase length of stay in the PACU would help determine more clearly the role of Xylocaine jelly use in the OR.

CHAPTER 59

Nursing Research Is for All Sorts of Nurses

Sally Rudy

More than 25 years ago, I worked in a position in which I collected data for research projects for a physician. The work piqued my interest in the many questions that could be answered by a study, but I was not involved in the study design, evaluation, or writing of those works at all. Somewhat grateful to be free of those academic responsibilities of which I knew little, I did not give it much thought as I turned my attention away from work and focused on family.

As the years passed, I knew that I wanted to continue with my education but made slow progress while working the minimal part-time hours. As my children grew, I began to think about returning to work to help pay for college expenses. Wanting more flexibility than I thought I could get with bedside nursing, I fell into a job in a simulation lab because someone was needed to work on a research project long left unfinished. Not really understanding the expectations of helping with an old research project that no one had time for, I charged ahead with a fearfully small amount of knowledge about research. Having always thought about teaching and research, it seemed like a good fit— no firm schedule, no time clocks, no off-hours, and yet, autonomy. I could wing the research project, right?

The problem became quite evident: Although I had the nursing knowledge, I did not have the education that I needed to teach or pursue research. I quickly enrolled in courses to complete my BSN and then continued on with graduate work. The real beauty in the process became clear as I was able to use my current studies all along the way in my position as an educator (and part-time newbie researcher) in the simulation lab. Both teaching and research opportunities grew as I worked with several helpful mentors along the way— accomplished researchers and authors from both medicine and nursing.

Fearful as I was about becoming more involved in research on my own ("You want me to do what?"), these mentors patiently guided me through the entire process, from institutional review board (IRB) and grant applications to basic idea, to outline, to final paper (after many rewrites, of course). That old research project was finally published in a nursing journal 6 years later. Although I did have a great deal of help with that first project, it was a seminal moment for me; I could do this! However, in the back of my mind was a nagging voice that kept asking if I wanted to go through such a protracted process again.

I stifled the voice and chose another personal topic of interest, one that is relevant to nursing education, professional development, and simulation education. I thought I was going to prove to the world that simulation was the key to teaching critical thinking! Everyone in the worlds of nursing and medical education and simulation wanted to know what I wanted to prove. I received a grant of $2,400 from an in-house service organization, the Association of Family and Friends, to fund the work. It was the perfect first grant to write because it was not complicated or long. The IRB approval process was likewise a good starter application; it qualified as exempt because of its educational focus. So, I chose a convenient study population that included all the new graduate nursing hires for the summer of 2006. They were a captive audience and would surely be interested in advancing nursing and simulation knowledge. How much easier could it get? I had those statistics and research courses under my belt and was on my way to academia fame.

I realized quickly that a meticulous study design was paramount and that I still had much to learn about conducting a research project. My final participants numbered only 30 after lofty dreams of nearly 100 eager new nurse subjects. I notified every nurse manager to ensure their support, and all my coworkers vowed to help when possible. Of course, I kept those mentors close at hand.

I completed the data collection after many glitches and much lost sleep, and I breathed a sigh of relief to be finally done. Although I still need to complete the manuscript, that sense of accomplishment could not be diminished. I knew that getting my feet wet was what I needed to do. Although many limitations arose in the study design, this project has become a pilot for a more definitive study that is now in development. Because my study group was smaller than expected, I have money left to continue the work under more controlled circumstances and with a modicum of wisdom gained. The project is being developed for the summer of 2008 with new-hire graduate nurses and cautious optimism.

I am buoyed by the enthusiasm and support of my coworkers and our nursing research department, and I hope to continue to share my experiences with the staff nurses who come to the simulation lab. Other study ideas materialize daily and will continue to inspire our research work in the simulation lab. Armed with a small amount of new knowledge from school and experience, I am encouraged to continue making a difference in the body of nursing research.

Acknowledgment: I would like to extend my warmest thanks to colleagues who have supported and mentored me along my research journey, particularly Bosseau Murray, Vicki Schirm, Lisa Sinz, Rosemary Polomano, and my nursing education coworkers.

A Pilot Program Using Simulation to Enhance Patient Education

Sally Rudy, MSN, RN

Purpose: Attention to promoting better decision-making by enhancing critical thinking skills of nurses is especially important in today's complex healthcare arena. High patient acuity, rapid technological advancements, reimbursement constraints, and staffing shortages all contribute to overwhelming pressure on newly graduated nurses. Research has shown that critical thinking skills can help new nurses facilitate learning and deal better with practice challenges. Research findings also suggest that promoting high-quality critical thinking skills among nurses can result in better patient care.

The goal of this project is to assess the efficacy of using simulation to teach critical thinking skills to new graduate nurses. In addition, we hope to better equip new graduate nurses to make sound clinical decisions by using critical thinking skills in the delivery of nursing care. Promoting critical thinking skills can enable nurses to better manage the usual everyday challenges of patient care and the more demanding crises that frequently occur in an academic medical center. Critical thinking allows for the timely, organized, and safer interpretation and integration of dynamic patient care information, thereby leading to improved patient care. The proposed study will use the innovative environment of the Simulation Development and Cognitive Science Laboratory at Penn State Hershey Medical Center to provide critical thinking skills training for new graduate nurses.

Design: A quasi-experimental design was used to conduct the study. All 30 study participants took the California Critical Thinking Skills Test (CCTST) initially. The group was randomly assigned to one of two groups, early and late training groups. The early training group then came to the simulation lab for three critical thinking sessions over a period of 2 months. Both groups then retook the CCTST, and the late training group was scheduled for critical thinking sessions in the simulation lab.

Methods: New graduate nurses were asked to give informed consent to participate in this project. Potential participants were 100 newly hired graduate nurses who began employment in the summer of 2006. Participants took a standardized critical thinking test (CCTST) during the first 2 weeks of orientation. They then participated in a series of small-group critical thinking exercises that pertained to common patient conditions encountered on their clinical unit. These scenarios took place in the simulation lab over a 2-to-3-month period. Upon completion of the critical thinking exercises, they were then asked to take the CCTST again. Nurse participant demographic data and results of the CCTST were analyzed to evaluate the nurses' critical thinking skills. Reports and accounts from participants were examined to provide a rich description of their experiences.

Results: No statistically significant differences were found in the CCTST scores before and after training using critical thinking exercises in the simulation lab. Participants did, however, find the sessions valuable. Most reported that they felt more confident in their beginning nursing practice. Several groups wanted further sessions.

Conclusions: The Penn State Hershey Simulation Development and Cognitive Science Laboratory provided a unique environment to systematically teach critical thinking skills to new graduate nurses during their orientation. This setting enabled nurses to experience "real-life" situations without fear of harming real patients. Using simulation to teach critical thinking skills has not been studied carefully because of the newness of the technology and the expense of the equipment. Patient simulation using high-fidelity manikins has only been used for the past 10 years in nursing education. Additional study is needed to assess the efficacy of using simulation to teach critical thinking skills. Clearly, better instruments for assessing critical thinking skills need to be developed or identified. This pilot has created an avenue for future research that might help to answer these questions. Evaluation and teaching of critical thinking skills in a simulation lab will allow timely feedback and ultimately provide new nurses with the requisite skills and knowledge to deliver high-quality patient care.

CHAPTER 60

I Teach, But Do I Reach?

Jean M. Mau

Several years ago, the mention of research raised connotations of academia—something that "others did," not something that a clinical nurse like me would ever consider. What does research have to do with my nursing practice? Then one day I was challenged with a question: Do you have any patients who are illiterate? How do you teach them? Do you reach them? I thought about this and realized that even though I took pride in presenting patients with the information I thought they needed, I did not check if they could read, understand the printed word. Did it make sense to them? You know the feeling that comes over you when you think that you have made an error? Well, that is the feeling that I had.

I am fortunate enough to be a part of a teaching institution that embraced the Health Literacy challenge: the ability to read, write, and understand basic healthcare information. I was part of a 1-month pilot study that was very successful. In fact, we were granted the 2005 Research of the Year Award from the Institute of Health Care Advancement for our work, "Impact of a Targeted Program Designed to Encourage Patients to Ask Questions Pertaining to Their Health: The Ask Me 3 Project."

I was so excited with our pilot results that we moved forward with a "real" research study. We wanted to explore patient teaching with nurses: *Would a set format encourage you to provide more patient education?* I applied for and successfully received a grant for funding. Then, the institutional review board—I really struggled with the formatting of the survey questions. We revised, revised, and revised until it was acceptable. It felt like an eternity, but in the end, our questions were more focused and would make the results more powerful. The two nursing units that participated were awesome; they really embraced the opportunity to participate in research and, as a result, provide even better patient care and education. The study lasted 3 months, and our outcomes spoke for themselves. We demonstrated not only a statistically significant increase in patient education provided by nurses but also increased patient satisfaction and decreased 30-day hospital readmission rates for patients with heart failure! The staff is eager to participate in more research. I am thrilled with the enthusiasm seen in the staff, and I was humbled by our results. The results have been showcased in our institution and in conferences in several states. Now, what should be our next study?

Based on my experience, I would find a mentor, a colleague to work with you. I learn best with the teach-back technique, or learning by example. This way, you can refocus if you get off track or if things do not go as you thought they would. Working with a multidisciplinary team is also helpful. In health care, we do not work in silos to provide quality care, so why would we do research in silos? My best advice is to try it; you may even be surprised and like it—and make a difference in someone's life!

Acknowledgments: I'd like to extend my warmest thanks to colleagues who have supported me on my research journey. Their encouragement and sense of humor helped me to take one step at a time and get through the entire research process in one piece!

Enhancing Nurse–Patient Communication Through "Ask Me 3"

Jean M. Mau, BS, MSN, RN, APN; and
Phyllis D. Wille, MS, RN, FNP-C, CNN

Background: Patient education is an essential component of nursing care. However, a lack of confidence in the ability to educate patients has been identified as a barrier for nurses in providing patient education.

Purpose: The scripted "Ask Me 3" questions assist nurses in providing clear, concise information that impacts patient education.

Methods: Ask Me 3, created by the Partnership for Clear Health Communication, was developed to promote clear communication between patient and provider. This program encourages patients to ask: (1) What is my main problem? (2) What do I need to do? and (3) Why is it important for me to do this? The answers to these questions help patients assume a more active partnership in their health care. Nurses (n = 31) received education on Ask Me 3. During the 3-month study period, nurses were encouraged to incorporate Ask Me 3 into all patient–nurse interactions. Pre- and postimplementation surveys were administered to evaluate different aspects of nurse–patient interactions. Patients with a diagnosis of heart failure (HF) (n = 126) were contacted postdischarge via the HF follow-up telephone call to evaluate patient education received.

Results: A paired t-test analysis demonstrated a statistically significant improvement in nurses' perceived ability ($p < .001$) to provide, and confidence ($p = .002$) in providing, patient education. Thirty-day readmission rates for HF decreased from 7.2% to less than 2.5% during the study period.

Conclusion: Nurses have an important role in helping patients understand and adhere to a therapeutic self-care plan. The Ask Me 3 format provides nurses with the confidence and ability to provide effective patient education. The decrease in readmissions for HF suggests an increase in patients' ability to understand the education and assume self-care posthospitalization. The significance seen in this study suggests that implementation of Ask Me 3 will foster increased collaboration between healthcare providers and patients in chronic care management, thereby decreasing the need for rehospitalization.

(November 2006–January 2007)

CHAPTER 61

Research: Something to Sink Your Teeth into

Stephanie A. Lopuszynski

Once upon a time, I was an admission nurse. Actually, I still am. I help direct patient care nurses to complete their paperwork and troubleshoot patient requests and problems at the bedside in my hospital. But I was looking for other ways to make a contribution in my institution, and one day I joined the ergonomics committee. This committee was investigating methods to increase caregiver safety in moving patients at the bedside (while also making it safer for the patients), and I thought this might be a project I could sink my teeth into.

I had no idea at the time that I was foreshadowing how the world of research was about to start nibbling on me! After 2 years of continuing in my admissions job and helping to bring a minimal lift program to Saint Joseph's Hospital of Atlanta, my director encouraged me to look into the nursing research council (NRC).

I met a very educated and enthusiastic nursing research director, but she also made me nervous. Any time I would speak with her, she used words or acronyms with which I was not very familiar—*SPSS, qualitative versus quantitative, IRB, abstract writing,* and others. And she always smiled knowingly as we became better acquainted, saying that someday I too would be doing some type of formal research study.

I shuddered at the thought. Research seemed like something that librarians from my past helped me to do when I was in school (more than a decade ago at this point). And although I respected our nursing research director, writing papers, collecting data, analyzing input, or anything related to those tasks sounded like a lot of hard work, late nights, and searching for an answer to research questions that I had not yet formulated!

By then, Saint Joseph's minimal lift program had passed its first year, and we discovered that we might have some research questions after all. After receiving a grant from the Robert Wood Johnson Foundation (RWJF), my hospital decided to study how to retain experienced nurses at the bedside, related to the minimal lift program.

The pressure was on! I had been working with our minimal lift program for its entire existence, and who better to advocate for it to the nursing staff (under the guise of research) than someone who truly wants the nursing staff to be safe? I had several conversations with our director of nursing research. Would I be alone, doing all the work for a research study with no one to guide me? Would I know what to do, where to look for resources, how to submit documents that made sense, how to work with the staff throughout the research process to accomplish our goals, or how to substantiate any theories about our minimal lift program? And, when it was all finished, how would I inform people of what I'd learned, and how would I apply those lessons to reality?

With a great deal of encouragement and mentoring from our nursing research director, I applied to conduct the research on Saint Joseph's minimal lift program. The main issue under consideration was the existence of a minimal lift program that had passed its "honeymoon phase" and the day-to-day challenges of sustaining a decrease in injuries to nurses (and other caregivers) that were related to patient movement. After a phenomenal decrease in lost work days, associated expenses, and injuries to bedside caregivers, the success of our minimal lift program was entering a new phase; the staff had to be reenergized to continue safe transfer and movement techniques for themselves and their patients, or there would be an increase in caregiver injury as complacency set in and people returned to "the way they have always done it."

At the same time, the world around us has changed; the average age of nurses at the bedside (depending on the journal you read) is 42–47 years old. And in approximately the next 10 years, this group of nurses is going to begin considering retirement. Many reasons are cited for this. One major theory is that after years of pushing, pulling, lifting, and moving the sicker, heavier, and less mobile hospital patients, nurses are leaving the bedside to pursue other, less back-aching, knee-twisting, shoulder-pulling options. Hospitals across the country—and philanthropic groups like the RWJF—recognize that ways must be found to encourage experienced nurses to remain in direct patient care. The unfortunate alternative is a much-reduced nursing workforce and even more potentially critical situations of safety at the bedside.

We needed someone who was willing to dig into this project wholeheartedly! With fingers crossed for luck, a lot of prayer, and hundreds of e-mails to my nursing research director, I plowed through the research landscape. Thousands of words were put to paper, institutional review board (IRB) and NRC approvals were acquired, hundreds of nursing staff surveys were completed, and hundreds of hours were spent working with nurses and other staff on educational and informational offerings encouraging the use of minimal lift equipment. Data were compiled, initial findings were presented, and final details were collected. I have now arrived at the point of writing up the research results and discussing the lessons we have learned!

Although much remains to be done to "finish our study," the feeling I now have about research has changed a bit. I don't shudder at the thought of conducting research. (Well, perhaps the shiver I get is not quite as severe anymore!) And although writing papers, collecting data, and analyzing input involve a lot of hard work, late nights, and searching for an answer to a research question, I have become a bit more enlightened. Research can be laborious because you must constantly explain to others why you are doing what you are doing, and what you hope to accomplish. Research can be mind- and office-pile-expanding because you must keep track of many little projects that are all part of the bigger picture at one time—and generate boxes of paperwork and/or computer files in the process.

Research can be frustrating as you discover the limitations of your schedule, study parameters, and your ability to finish all the things you really want to do, and then tie everything together to make all your efforts sensible to other people.

But research is intriguing because it allows you to satisfy your curiosity for figuring out why things work or don't work. Research allows you to see more clearly what may need to happen next for the project at hand. Research is satisfying, inspiring, and tantalizing because it takes you to other projects, questions, "what-ifs," and a buffet of other places that you may not have considered before. In essence, research can make you hungry to learn more and explore more about your profession. And that can be a very "tasty" thing.

Overcoming a fear or shudder at the mention of the words *research study* is like everything you have ever figured out about being a nurse. If there was a procedure (such as working with a tracheostomy patient, in my case) for which there was a great deal of trepidation, I overcame that by begging for help in working with such patients and dealing with all the issues with every single one who came onto my nursing unit when I worked at the bedside. And that is partly the same way I overcame the uncomfortable feelings I equated with doing research.

Step up to the question at hand, take one bite at a time, and ask a lot of questions (and pray for someone to work with you who has the heart and soul of a teacher). Then, put your hands on what needs to be done; work with it, revise it, and keep at it every day if necessary. There will come a time when, if research doesn't become a little tiny bit easier, it will at least become somewhat more doable and less scary. You may even find that you've accomplished something you can be very proud of—and walk away from your research study feeling that you have completed something from which others will benefit. And isn't that why we all entered nursing to begin with: to provide something to others that would make us feel that we were contributing to those around us? Research is perhaps something for you to consider. What will you sink your teeth into next?

Acknowledgment: I sincerely extend my heartfelt thanks, appreciation, and utmost respect to Dr. Diana Meeks-Sjostrom, whose terrific sense of humor, phenomenal encouragement, and endless energy were exactly what I needed to accomplish a great research study. You're the best!

Wisdom at Work: Retaining Experienced Nurses at the Bedside

Stephanie A. Lopuszynski, BSN, BS, RN

Purpose: This institutional review board-approved pilot study was conducted to acquire novel information regarding the bedside nurse's satisfaction with current in-house minimal lift equipment (MLE) and its use and to determine if these devices maintain or increase retention of experienced nurses at the bedside by reducing potential patient movement-related (PMR) injuries.

Design: A descriptive, exploratory study design was used to determine bedside nurses' satisfaction with, and level of, PMR usage of MLE pre- and postintervention.

Methods: A preintervention 15-item adapted survey was self-administered by 92 direct patient care nurses on any unit using MLE. Interventions, including hands-on facilitation of MLE at the patient bedside, unit-based MLE in-services, key employee training, and other educational and informational offerings were presented. At approximately 4 weeks postintervention, the same satisfaction survey was readministered to 88 nurses on the same nursing units that participated in the preintervention survey.

Results: Bedside nurses want more instruction, encouragement, and management support for using MLE and will more likely use MLE if they have enough devices and accessibility to them to assist their patients. Additionally, the integration of a minimal lift program into a hospital's culture must be ongoing in order to sustain and build on improvements to nurses' PMR injury rates and to further realize retention of experienced RNs at the bedside.

Conclusions: By determining the relationship between the nurse's satisfaction with, and usage of, the MLE and years of experience of the nurse, additional facilitated initiatives can be developed to decrease the number of PMR injuries to bedside nurses. These initiatives will assist in enhancing and improving the retention of experienced RNs at the bedside for the target hospital and any other healthcare facility undertaking minimal lift programs. The results of this research may also lay the foundation for future interventional studies related to decreasing PMR injuries using MLE.

(2007)

CHAPTER 62

Recitation of a Research Novice: A Staff Development Perspective

Carol Korman

Although my MSN program had prepared me for research through writing a thesis, 12 years had passed since I had taken on this big endeavor. It took that long, I think, to get over the exasperation that comes from having to "jump through the hoops" of conducting a study. I thought I knew what I was getting into: write, rewrite, calculate, and exasperate! It had been a long time since my days of graduate school. However, as an education coordinator in charge of a career ladder program, I knew that the only way to really evaluate a program was through quantitative survey to ascertain both the positive and the negative perceptions of those nurses who were working so hard to provide practice exemplars to highlight their career accomplishments. With a lot of encouragement from my director, I embarked on this journey again, fully knowing that the road ahead would not be easy—but few big accomplishments are ever easy.

OK, I remember from my days in grad school several things about beginning a research study. Test your idea with the "So what?" question. I wanted to measure satisfaction with the career ladder. I wanted to see if it was actually doing what it should be doing: rewarding and recognizing registered nurses by measuring their practice with theoretical standards based on experiential practice evidence. OK, it passed the "So what?" test. This was important because the ladder program is quite a costly endeavor for the hospital.

The next thing I remembered from grad school was the need to find a valid and reliable tool that can stand up to rigorous statistical testing if I wanted to someday get the study published and present it at conferences. So I hit the literature and found only two actual tools that were pertinent to career ladders. Most of the articles merely described clinical ladder programs and their content; though interesting, this was not an evidence-based review of whether the ladders were doing what they were supposed to be doing: increasing job satisfaction and rewarding the registered nurse for expertise in action. Along with that, our ladder was unique in that it had three tracks: clinical, education, and management. An educator or manager could participate along with the clinical nurses. Yes, I really needed to do this study. I called the nurse who had formulated the tool and began to establish a networking relationship that led to meeting her in person at a national conference.

I also remembered to always consult a statistician before starting to formulate the project design. Oops—that takes money! I applied for small grants through my hospital and through a local chapter of Sigma Theta Tau and received both, so the statistician was consulted. Talk about walking through mud to decipher the statistical intricacies of quantitative research!

Lastly, I remembered from my grad school days that the process is much less painful if you have someone to work with who is knowledgeable in nursing research. So I asked my director, who has a PhD in nursing, if she would like to be my coinvestigator, and she happily agreed. As principal investigator, I was responsible for the study, from the institutional review board approval through organizing the process. I used my director primarily as a consultant because her schedule was already tight with her position responsibilities. Little did I know the arduous task that would ensue for the next 3 years (yes, I said 3 years!). Make sure you get along well with your coinvestigator, especially if he or she is more the expert at conducting research. Don't take the coinvestigator's comments personally; he or she only wants your success in the study, which at times means you have to write, rewrite, write again, and then wait. Oh yes, that was the other item I had forgotten from grad school, but it really hit home: Make sure you love the topic you are going to research. You will eat, sleep, and breathe it until you are finished. Yes, I have thoroughly digested it now and can talk about it in my sleep (and have talked about it in my sleep, according to my husband!). Once your research is completed, you are the expert of your content.

My study is complete and is now in the dissemination phase. What are the best things for me that came about through doing the research? I've won a national award for conducting professional development research. I've presented and networked with numerous nurses at conferences about career ladders, and I get numerous e-mails of inquiry about our three-track ladder. I have renewed my knowledge of the research process and the importance of working with statisticians from the idea phase through data analysis, and I have gained a high respect for their working knowledge of statistics. I am not the statistical expert, yet I am growing in my knowledge of this area thanks to those who have helped me correlate the numbers with the reality of the program. I am currently writing a manuscript to submit for publication, with the help of a professor of nursing from a neighboring university. My research will not be complete until it is published. This challenge has also appeared in my dreams (the many aspects of writing a research manuscript are sometimes quite invasive to the psyche). Was it worth it? You bet. Was it easy? No way. But remember, great accomplishments are never easy.

Acknowledgment: I'd like to acknowledge the expertise of my coinvestigator, Aris Eliades, PhD, RN, for the guidance she provided to me as a novice researcher. I'd like to extend my warmest thanks to Kristine Gill, PhD, RN, who continues to mentor my writing endeavors, and to Rose Baker, PhD, MSN, (c), APRN, BC, my role model of professionalism and kindness.

Program Evaluation of a Career Ladder for Registered Nurses

Carol Korman, MSN, RN, BC

Background: Human resources executives report that the most effective retention tactic is providing career advancement opportunities to nurses. With nationwide nursing shortages, it is timely to refocus on the role of career ladders as a retention tool. Studies of clinical ladders are present in the literature, but little literature exists about career ladders in nursing.

Purpose: This study evaluates a career ladder for registered nurses. The career ladder studied comprises three tracks and is designed to recognize and reward registered nurses who demonstrate expertise in the areas of clinical, education, and management.

Design and Methods: A descriptive study design was employed to survey registered nurse participants in a career ladder program at a freestanding children's hospital in the Midwest. Data were collected within a 1-month period via online survey. A 22-item instrument with a Likert scale and a Cronbach's alpha of 0.95 was modified for this study. A total of 136 nurses completed the survey, for a return rate of 78%.

Results: The modified research instrument was found to be reliable with a Cronbach's alpha of 0.92. Nurses with an MSN degree had the highest overall total scores on the instrument, and BSN-prepared nurses had the lowest scores. However, a statistically significant difference was not found between levels of educational preparation. The findings indicate that nurses had the opportunities to acquire the knowledge, skills, and activities to meet the career ladder criteria; the career ladder allowed nurses to choose a level of involvement in nursing activities; career ladder expectations were reviewed so that participants clearly understood expectations; evaluation was fair and equitable; and advancement in the career ladder provided a sense of accomplishment and professional satisfaction about their nursing career. The findings also indicated that career ladder participants did not believe that advancement was valued by nursing colleagues. Analysis of data by track revealed that nurses in the education track had the highest overall scores, nurses in the management track had the lowest overall scores, and nurses who advanced on the clinical track had higher scores compared with advancement on the education or management track.

Conclusions: A 78% completion return rate for the survey demonstrates the efficacy of nurses completing a survey online. The instrument used in this study is a reliable tool for evaluation of a career or clinical ladder. Educational preparation did not impact the scores. Participation in a career ladder allows nurses at any level of educational preparation, from diploma to PhD, to demonstrate professional development. Decreased scores for participants in the management track may be reflective of an evolving leadership role versus management role within the institution. The results of this study provide empirical data for revision of the career ladder program and address a gap in the literature by providing data for evaluating a career ladder in nursing.

CHAPTER 63

The Power of Team Research

Lisa Williams,
Deborah Morehouse, Christina Lloyd,
Dena McCoy, and Elizabeth Miller

This is a story about the power of team research. This story represents our personal journey about the fears we overcame and the unique skills, talents, and contributions that each of us brought to the table in developing a strong, successful, and productive research team.

We are five neonatal intensive care unit (NICU) nurses with 3–20 years of clinical nursing experience but little experience in research. Our story began when we identified the need to conduct research as members of our NICU Shared Nursing Leadership Resource & Innovation Council. As a team, over 18 months, we identified our nursing research problem, developed our research protocol entitled "Neonatal Thermoregulation Throughout the Perioperative Experience," gained all hospital and institutional review board (IRB) approvals, and were funded by an intramural grant. We are now in the phase of data collection. The following vignettes tell our story.

Nurse Investigator Lisa: As an experienced NICU nurse and leader in my unit, I had long recognized the need for nursing research but also felt that this was an area of weakness for most NICU nurses, including myself. I felt a responsibility to help advance nursing research but wasn't sure where to begin. Although I could imagine dozens of clinical questions that were worth exploring, I lacked the experience necessary to lead such a project. During the course of a regular management operations meeting, a special guest was introduced—someone who was hired for the sole purpose of mentoring nursing research. I contacted the research mentor immediately. We agreed that the first meeting with the mentor was a worthwhile venture, but I am certain that no one in the group anticipated the work that was to come. Neither did we anticipate the professional satisfaction that would come with the experience.

As I look back over the process, I was most nervous about producing a worthwhile product, one that added to the scientific body of knowledge and was useful to our own unit. It was difficult to be confident about researching a clinical problem because we had never done so before. This fear dissipated

331

with each group meeting as we were mentored to use our individual skills and expertise to accomplish our work. Although I could not claim a leadership role in developing a research proposal, I was able to lead the group in other ways. Facilitating cooperation among my coinvestigators was extremely important, as was helping them stay focused and on task when we all were faced with competing priorities. I was also instrumental in connecting the group with the resources and contacts that were required along the way.

Although we are far from finished, it is difficult to describe the sense of pride and accomplishment for what we have achieved. Our protocol, which was IRB approved, and the subsequent research grant we were awarded represent an amazing product of group collaboration that far surpasses anything that we had imagined when we set out on this journey. I am thrilled to have gained this experience and am confident that I will be exploring more clinical questions that I had previously contemplated but had no idea how to approach. I am grateful to be working with a group who is so committed and eager to learn and with a mentor who not only showed us the ropes but also gave us exactly the right amount of guidance and encouragement to move us along.

Nurse Investigator Christina: My fears of doing nursing research—and taking on the principal investigator role for our study—spanned the typical spectrum of not knowing the research process to being weary of the work and time commitments required to do a quality scientific study. When the opportunity arose to work with a dedicated nursing research mentor, the first fear was virtually eradicated. However, the second fear—the amount of work and time commitment—was amplified. I laugh now as I think back to one of our first meetings with our mentor, who said, "Christina, you are going to know my cell phone number by heart when we are done with this." I amicably nodded, silently thinking, *What have I got myself into now?* Well, she was right; I do know her cell phone number by heart, but the fear of time commitment to this project has definitely been eased. She taught me how to push forward during certain critical deadline weeks, staying at work late into the night and then taking time to reenergize during other less demanding weeks.

I have learned how a strong team functions to get work done by fostering every member's strengths and passion. I also value the many interdisciplinary colleagues I have met during this journey and their contributions to the research process. I have no doubt that this will not be the last time I work with my new colleagues in biostatistics, research, grants management, the IRB, ethics, and in other various hospital leadership positions. I think the main attribute I have brought to our research team is organization. By keeping us on track for deadlines, we were motivated to push ahead when the workload seemed daunting. I also believe that I brought a sense "for the big picture." I tend to step back from details and visualize how things will ultimately fit together, while learning from team members who are detail oriented. Research for the individual nurse can seem like a distant professional goal, but as a member of a research team, the goal is right in reach.

Nurse Investigator Elizabeth: When I joined this team, I had a little over 1 year of nursing experience, so it was a bit overwhelming to be surrounded with so much experience and talent. I considered my coinvestigators to be the best and the brightest at our institution and questioned how I would fit in and be an equal with these smart and remarkable nurses. I feared not living up to their standards and looking "dumb" because I had no experience with research. At times, I also felt overwhelmed because innovative ideas and critical evaluation pertaining to our research came so easily to them, but not to me.

After spending 2 months on the team, I realized that my fears were unfounded. My team members, although still the best and the brightest, had as little research experience as I did. I was treated as an equal partner. They expected me to pull equal weight. I loved the challenge. I felt like an equal for the first time in my nursing career. Having recently completed nursing school in this age of PowerPoint presentations and online classes, one particular talent that I brought to my team was my computer knowledge. I led the initiative to configure our data collection tool, decipher "computer" glitches in the many documents we produced, and develop a poster presentation of our work for our annual research day. During my last 3 years as a nurse, being part of this team has helped me grow the most and demonstrated to me the true power of nursing.

Nurse Researcher Dena: If someone had told me a year ago that I would grow to love nursing research, I would have laughed. Until 18 months ago, I did not participate in nursing research beyond using findings from others to inform my practice. There just did not seem to be enough time in the day to conduct research. The entire research process seemed overwhelming, and it was difficult to know where to begin. That was until the chair of our resource and innovation council mentioned the possibility of engaging in a research project and challenged another NICU council to a race to publication. The motivation of a little healthy competition was just what I needed.

As I listened on the unit, it became clear that my nurse colleagues felt that our babies were having negative outcomes related to perioperative hypothermia. Our council discussed this issue and concluded that it required further investigation. I led the collection of preliminary data that supported the assertion that a clinical problem existed. Fueled by a desire to improve the clinical problem, our team proceeded to develop a research proposal. While we worked on our study, my team members constantly amazed me. Their passion for our patients never wavered, and together we put together a research protocol that exceeded anything that we could have done individually. I realize that I had fears about nursing research because I did not understand the impact of a high-performing team. I thought that all the work was a burden to be carried by one person. Now I know that working with a great team minimizes the burdens and amplifies the joys of nursing research.

Nurse Investigator Debbie: If you had asked me about my fears 18 months ago, before we began our nursing research project, my response would have been very different than it is today. The idea of nursing research was exciting, intriguing, and a new adventure—like traveling to a foreign country. Yet, when traveling to a foreign land, you don't simply buy a ticket and go. You have to do your homework, plan the details, work out itineraries, buy a book to help with understanding the language, learn some of the language, choose your traveling companions, hire a guide, plan a budget, and apply for special visa approval before you begin your journey. The excitement of the trip far outweighs any fears you might have, and you plunge right into the adventure. The nursing research journey is not unlike traveling to foreign territories. It involves a foreign culture with a foreign language and foreign customs. You would be lost without a guide.

After 18 months, the initial excitement has been replaced with a little travel fatigue but also a great appreciation for this new culture. The traveling companions and guides have made the experience incredible. We have a gang mentality, with strength in numbers, and no fear as a group. The energy supplied by some members of the group continuously revitalizes other members—when one wanes, the other surges. As a bedside nurse, I am on the frontline. I see the data collection in real time. This is motivation. Any fears that I have are truly insignificant when I envision the potential benefits our study may have for our babies. The journey is not over, but it has been a great adventure thus far.

Postscript: During the course of this study, three of the coauthors have enrolled in a master's program.

Neonatal Thermoregulation Throughout the Perioperative Experience

Lisa Williams, BSN, RN;
Deborah Morehouse, MSN, RN; Christina Lloyd, MS, RNC;
Dena McCoy, BSN, RN; and Elizabeth Miller, BSN, RN

Purpose: Neonates admitted to the neonatal intensive care unit (NICU) often require surgical intervention. Maintaining normothermia is a major concern because hypothermia is associated with significant morbidity, yet a substantial gap in the literature exists related to negative sequelae of neonatal perioperative hypothermia. As NICU nurses, we observed the occurrence of postoperative hypothermia. In a preliminary study of 31 normothermic neonates undergoing procedures in the operating room (OR), 18 (58%) returned hypothermic postoperatively, and all 5 undergoing surgery in the NICU remained normothermic (relative risk = 2.17, p = 0.0013). These findings warranted further investigation. Therefore, the aims of this study are to describe neonatal perioperative thermal instability and identify where (OR, NICU) and when it occurs (pre-, intra-, and/or postoperatively).We will also describe and quantify the adverse cardiovascular, respiratory, and metabolic outcomes and associated diagnostic tests and support interventions of neonates who develop perioperative hypothermia versus those who do not.

Design: Descriptive-comparative.

Methods: We will include 96 neonates admitted to the NICU who are sequentially scheduled for an operative procedure in the OR (48 infants) or NICU (48 infants). Existing data from the bedside record will be collected about temperatures and frequency of adverse cardiovascular, respiratory, and metabolic outcomes during the pre-, intra-, and postoperative periods, and associated diagnostic tests and support interventions during the intra- and postoperative periods. Analyses will examine the relative risks and proportional differences in rates of hypothermia and adverse outcomes across the perioperative phases, as well as the relative risks and proportional differences in rates of diagnostic tests and support interventions in the intra- and postoperative phases between neonates who become hypothermic and those who do not.

Results and Conclusions: This study is currently nearing the end of data collection. The long-term objective is to determine whether corrective interventions are required to optimize the neonate's ability to remain normothermic regardless of the operative setting. This study will bridge the literature gap by documenting whether a problem exists, where and when it exists, and to what extent. If thermal instability is identified, corrective interventions focused on the points of care will be identified and evaluated in Phase 2. The processes we use likely will be useful to other pediatric institutions who also may confront perioperative neonatal thermal instability and who wish to investigate this issue.

Note: This study has been funded by Children's Research Institute, Children's National Medical Center, Washington, DC.

Frequently Asked Questions (FAQs) About Nursing Research

The following questions are often asked by nurses who are new to research or who have a fear that they can't do research. Our response to that is, yes you can!

Q: What is research?
Research is a "systematic inquiry that uses orderly, disciplined methods to answer questions or solve problems" (Polit & Beck, 2008, p. 765).

Three types of research are basic research, applied research, and clinical research.

Q: What is basic research?
This is "research designed to extend the base of knowledge in a discipline for the sake of knowledge production of theory construction, rather than for solving an immediate problem" (Polit & Beck, 2008, p. 748).

Q: What is applied research?
This is "research designed to find a solution to an immediate practical problem" (Polit & Beck, 2008, p. 765).

Q: What is clinical research?
This is "research designed to generate knowledge to guide nursing practice" (Polit & Beck, 2008, p. 749).

Q: What is EBP?
EBP stands for evidence-based practice. EBP is "a practice that involves making clinical decisions on the best available evidence with an emphasis on evidence from disciplined research" (Poit & Beck, 2008, p. 753).

Q: What's the difference between PI and nursing research?

That is a great question and an issue that often needs to be clarified. *PI* refers to *performance improvement* and is usually associated with improving the performance on a specific nursing unit (internally), not necessarily improving performance elsewhere. In some hospitals, PI projects do not require approval by the institutional review board (IRB), whereas in other hospitals, it is required. Research is a systematic inquiry that uses disciplined methods to answer questions or solve problems. Often, a goal of research is for the findings to be generalizable—that is, that the findings from the study can be applicable from one sample to a population. Research studies do require IRB review and/or approval. Remember to check with your organization before you begin the research process so that you know your organization's research requirements.

Q: Why do nurses want to do research?

Because it is a growing expectation of professional nurses at all levels, especially if your hospital has Magnet designation. As professionals, it is our responsibility to ensure that our nursing practice is evidence based and that conducting research generates new knowledge to guide our nursing practice. (Think of it as learning a new skill that will advance your knowledge and expertise *and* contribute to improving the quality of patient and nursing care!)

Q: Do I need an advanced degree to do research?

No. However, if you are a research novice, you will need the expertise of a research mentor and other experts to assist you on your research journey. Contact your nursing education department to find out what resources your hospital has available to help you.

Q: Do I need any special training to conduct research?

Yes. It is federal law that all researchers complete a human subjects training program to learn about protecting the rights of human subjects involved in research. Check with your organization's IRB for the specific program that must be completed prior to conducting a study. You can also access human subjects training at http://phrp.nihtraining.com/users/login.php.

In addition, the National Institute for Nursing Research (NINR) has a free online research training program for developing nurse scientists at http://www.nursescientists.com/.

Q: Will doing research help me to advance in my job?

We certainly hope so! Many hospitals now include research as part of the requirements for nurse advancement. Check with your organization for specifics.

Q: Will I get paid to do research?
That is another great question! Payment for your time and effort will depend on your organization. Many hospitals provide compensation for research-related activities, so be sure to check with your supervisor.

Q: How do I get started?
First, meet with your nursing unit manager(s) and let them know of your interest. They will discuss your topic with you and decide if it is a priority for the unit/hospital and suggest that you meet with the director of nursing research or the person designated at your hospital to help you on the research journey.

Q: Is there anybody within my hospital to help me do the research?
Many hospitals have multiple resources to help you, such as librarians, statisticians, nurse researchers, grant writers, and editors. Check with your nursing education department to identify what resources are available. If there are none internally, check with a college of nursing at a nearby university. Also refer to the list of nursing research resources found elsewhere in this book.

Q: Are there any special forms or templates that I can use to help me?
Check with your nursing education or staff development department because many of them have forms and templates specific to their organization. If they don't have any specific forms for nursing research, obtain a nursing research textbook from the library. One example of a comprehensive textbook that includes multiple forms and templates is *Nursing Research: Generating and Assessing Evidence for Nursing Practice* by Polit and Beck (2008).

Q: How do I know what type of study to do?
It depends on your research question and how the data will be collected. Check with your director of nursing research and/or biostatistician to assist you with this.

Q: Where can I find studies related to my specialty?
A quick and easy method is to contact your national nursing specialty organization to see what studies are in their archives. You can also do a literature search to see what has been published on your topic of interest and in your specialty.

Q: Why do I need to do a literature review?
A review of the literature helps to identify what has already been studied on a topic and any gaps that may lead to future research opportunities.

Q: What about statistics? Is there anyone to help me with that?
Yes! Nurses are not trained to be statisticians. Check with educators at your hospital because many of them may collaborate with biostatisticians. If you

don't find anyone there, check with a local college of nursing. Many of them have faculty who teach statistics courses and who may be available to help you. Remember, it is important to discuss your research question and data collection methods with a statistician *before* you begin the process!

Q: What is the IRB?
IRB stands for *institutional review board.* This is a formal committee with protocols to review research plans. The duty of the IRB is to protect the rights of human subjects and uphold ethical principles. Some hospitals may call this committee a human subjects review board (HSRB) or something similar.

Q: How do I write a research proposal?
A proposal usually includes the following: problem statement, research question/hypotheses, literature review, framework, sample, population, methods, and data analysis. The IRB has specific forms that ask questions about your research study; these questions easily will be answered by your proposal.

Q: How do I know what forms to fill out for the IRB?
Check with your IRB to determine which forms best meet the criteria for your study. Many of these are now available online through hospital Web sites.

Q: How can I get my study published?
First, you need to decide where you would like to see it published. Next, you need to contact the editor or send a query to that publication to determine the criteria for manuscript. Then, just do it!

Q: How can I make a professional poster presentation for a conference?
Check with the educators in your hospital for assistance. Those hospitals affiliated with universities may have a digital imaging division with experts who may also provide assistance. Fees for this may vary but are often paid by the nursing division if the poster will be used at a professional conference.

Q: Are funds available to pay for my research studies?
Some hospitals have nursing research funds or other designated funds to assist nurses with their research studies. If not, check with your hospital's foundation and development person; these people are often aware of alternative funding resources. In addition, check online for grant funding availability from your specialty and other organizations. A few examples of sites to check for funding are:

- The American Association of Critical-Care Nurses: http://www.aacn.org
- Sigma Theta Tau: http://www.nursingsociety.org
- The Robert Wood Johnson Foundation: http://www.rwjf.org

- The National Institutes for Nursing Research (NINR): http://www.ninr.nih
  .gov/ResearchAndFunding/DEA/OEP/FundingOpportunities/default.htm

REFERENCES

Polit, D. F., & Beck, C. T. (2008). *Nursing research: Generating and assessing evidence for nursing practice* (8th ed.). Philadelphia: Wolters Kluwer/Lippincott Williams & Wilkins.

Glossary

Abstract: A brief description of a completed or proposed study, usually located at the beginning of a report or proposal.

Analysis: The process of organizing and synthesizing data so as to answer research questions and test hypotheses.

Anonymity: Protection of participants' confidentiality such that even the researcher cannot link individuals with information provided.

Applied research: Research designed to find a solution to an immediate practical problem.

Basic research: Research designed to extend the base of knowledge in a discipline for the sake of knowledge production of theory construction rather than to solve an immediate problem.

Clinical research: Research designed to generate knowledge to guide nursing practice.

Consent form: A written agreement signed by a study participant and a researcher concerning the terms and conditions of voluntary participation in a study.

Data: The pieces of information obtained in a study.

Data analysis: The systematic organization and synthesis of research data and, in quantitative studies, the testing of hypotheses using those data.

Data collection: The formal process of collection of data in a standardized fashion.

Eligibility criteria: The criteria designating the specific attributes of the target population, by which people are selected for inclusion in a study.

Evidence-based practice (EBP): A practice that involves making clinical decisions on the best available evidence, with an emphasis on evidence from disciplined research.

Institutional review board (IRB): A group of individuals from an institution who convene to review proposed and ongoing studies with respect to ethical considerations.

Instrument: The device used to collect data (e.g., a questionnaire, test, or observation schedule).

Journal club: A group that meets regularly in clinical settings to discuss and critique research reports that appear in journals.

Literature review: A critical summary of research on a topic of interest, often prepared to put a research problem in context.

Nursing research: Systemic inquiry designed to develop knowledge about issues of importance to the nursing profession.

Outcomes research: Research designed to document the effectiveness of healthcare services and the end results of patient care.

PICOT: An acronym that stands for: P—patient, problem, or population; I—intervention; C—comparison; O—outcome; T—time (timeline).

Reliability: The degree of consistency or dependability with which an instrument measures an attribute.

Replication: The deliberate repetition of research procedures in a second investigation for the purpose of determining if earlier results can be confirmed.

Research: Systematic inquiry that uses orderly, disciplined methods to answer questions or solve problems.

Research methods: The techniques used to structure a study and to gather and analyze information in a systematic fashion.

Research problem: An enigmatic or perplexing condition that can be investigated through disciplined inquiry.

Research question: A statement of the specific query that the researcher wants to answer to address a research problem.

Research utilization: The use of some aspect of a study in an application unrelated to the original research.

Response rate: The rate of participation in a study, calculated by dividing the number of persons participating by the number of persons sampled.

Results: The answers to research questions, obtained through an analysis of the collected data.

Sample: A subset of a population selected to participate in a study.

Statistical analysis: The organization and analysis of quantitative data using statistical procedures, including both descriptive and inferential statistics.

Statistical significance: A term indicating that the results from an analysis of sample data are unlikely to have been caused by chance, at a specified level of probability.

Systematic review: A rigorous and systematic synthesis of research findings on a common or strongly related question.

Validity: A quality criterion referring to the degree to which inferences made in a study are accurate and well-founded; in measurement, the degree to which an instrument measures what it is intended to measure.

REFERENCES

Polit, D. F., & Beck, C. T. (2008). *Nursing research: Generating and assessing evidence for nursing practice* (8th ed.). Philadelphia: Wolters Kluwer/Lippincott Williams & Wilkins.

Online Nursing Research Resources

National Institute for Nursing Research (NINR)

http://www.nih.gov/ninr

Promotes and supports clinical and basic research to establish a scientific basis for the care of individuals across the life span and illness trajectory, and for the promotion of healthy lifestyles, quality of life in those with chronic illness, and care for individuals at the end of life.

Eastern Nursing Research Society (ENRS)

http://www.enrs-go.org

Provides a forum for nurse researchers in the northeastern United States to promote and support regional nursing research, stimulate interest in scientific inquiry, and promote evidence-based nursing practice.

Midwest Nursing Research Society (MNRS)

http://www.mnrs.org

Purpose is to support, encourage, and improve the quality of nursing research within the region through networking, provision of dissemination avenues, and promotion of resources.

Western Institute of Nursing (WIN)

http://www.ohsu.edu/son/win

Western regional nursing organization that brings together a diverse community of nurses in a shared commitment to nursing research that enhances practice.

Southern Nursing Research Society (SNRS)
http://www.snrs.org
Organization serving the southern region that endeavors to advance nursing research, promote dissemination and utilization of research findings, facilitate the career development of nurses and nursing students as researchers, and enhance communication.

Sigma Theta Tau International (SITTI)
http://www.nursingsociety.org
Nursing honor society dedicated to improving the health of people worldwide by increasing the scientific base of nursing practice; funds research projects.

Location and Bed Size
Demographics of Represented
Magnet Hospitals

Thirty-one Magnet hospitals are represented by the stories told in this book. The location and bed size demographics related to these hospitals are shown in Table Demo-1 and Table Demo-2.

Table Demo-1   Location of Represented Magnet Hospitals

Urban setting	11 hospitals
Suburban setting	9 hospitals
Town/city	8 hospitals
Rural	3 hospitals

Table Demo-2   Location of Represented Magnet Hospitals

Fewer than 300 beds	9 hospitals
300–500 beds	9 hospitals
500–1000 beds	11 hospitals
More than 1000 beds	2 hospitals

Future Trends of Nursing Research

ONCOLOGY NURSING SOCIETY

The Oncology Nursing Society (ONS) is a professional organization of more than 35,000 registered nurses and other healthcare providers dedicated to excellence in patient care, education, research, and administration in oncology nursing. The mission of ONS is to promote excellence in oncology nursing and quality cancer care.

Beginning in 1980, approximately every four years, ONS has surveyed its members to determine the society's research priorities. In 2004, an electronic survey was administered to a random sample of the general ONS membership (N = 2205) and all ONS members in the United States with doctoral degrees (N = 627). The respondents (n = 431, response rate 15%) were asked to rate each of the 117 topics using a 5-point Likert scale in reference to the question, "How important is it to conduct new research in each of the following topics?" The top ten research priorities identified by the survey are 1) quality of life; 2) participation in decision making about treatment in advanced disease; 3) patient and family education; 4) participation in decision making about treatment; 5) pain; 6) tobacco use and exposure; 7) screening and early detection of cancer; 8) prevention of cancer and cancer risk reduction; 9) palliative care; and 10) evidence-based practice (Berger et al., 2005).

The ONS research agenda informs the ONS leadership, membership, and individuals and groups outside the organization about the scientific priorities of the ONS membership. It is developed through a consensus-building process of ONS nurse scientists, advanced practice nurses, and a consumer, and is reviewed, evaluated, and revised at 2-year intervals. The development of the 2005–2009 ONS research agenda was guided by the 2004 ONS Research Priorities Survey results, priority research areas of other cancer and nursing research funding organizations, and the review of the state of the science of oncology nursing research. Priority research content areas identified by the agenda are 1) cancer symptoms and side effects; 2) individual and family-focused psychosocial and behavioral research; 3) health promotion: primary and secondary prevention; 4) late effects of cancer treatment and long-term survivorship issues for patients and their families; 5) nursing-sensitive patient outcomes; and 6) translational research. All populations are relevant for study for all of the content areas including populations across the lifespan, families and caregivers, and vulnerable populations in relation to health disparities in minority groups of all types (ONS, 2007).

Nursing practice based on scientific evidence is essential for delivering quality cancer care. Nursing research addressing the ONS research priorities will provide scientific evidence for nursing practice and will impact patient outcomes. ONS and the ONS Foundation support oncology nurses in conducting research. Research funding for oncology nursing research is available from the ONS Foundation (http://www.ons.org/awards).

Linda Eaton, MN, RN, AOCN
Oncology Nursing Society
Pittsburgh, PA

REFERENCES

Berger, A., Berry, D., Christopher, K., Greene, A., Maliski, S., Swenson, K., et al. (2005). Oncology Nursing Society year 2004 research priorities survey. *Oncology Nursing Forum*, 32(2), 281–290.

Oncology Nursing Society. (2007). *Research Agenda & Priorities—Research Agenda*. Retrieved February 28, 2008, from http://www.ons.org/research/information/agenda.shtml

AMERICAN ASSOCIATION OF NEUROSCIENCE NURSES

A review of neuroscience nursing research from 1960 to 1988 identified the following trends: 1) an increase in the number of studies; 2) a shift from chronic to acute care; 3) a focus on physiological variables; 4) a slight trend toward theory; and, 5) a utilization of more complex methodology. Trends seen from 1989 to 2000 include 1) a continued increase in the number of studies; 2) a focus on neurological populations (i.e., multiple sclerosis, stroke, and epilepsy); 3) a focus on chronic illness and psychosocial variables; 4) a continued trend toward theory; and 5) a use of complex research methods.

Prevention has remained a gap in neuroscience nursing research for the past 40 years. A strong need exists to test nursing interventions with associated patient outcomes. Patient populations requiring investigation include the elderly and other neurological conditions such as amyotrophic lateral sclerosis (ALS). Health disparities exist in many health-related conditions, and neuroscience is no exception, yet we lack appreciation and understanding of this reality. Efforts need to be directed toward development of instruments to measure phenomena of concern for neuroscience nurses. Finally, these gaps could be addressed through renewed collaboration between academia and hospital-based nurse researchers.

Susan Fowler, PhD, RN, CNRN, FAHA
American Association of Neuroscience Nurses
Glenview, IL

Submitted by Colleen DiIorio, PhD, RN, FAAN, Professor, Emory University, Rollins School of Public Health—Neuroscience Nursing Foundation (NNF) Special Lecturer 2007; Susan B. Fowler, PhD, RN, CNRN, FAHA, President, American Association of Neuroscience Nurses 2007–2008

ACADEMY OF MEDICAL-SURGICAL NURSES

The Academy of Medical-Surgical Nurses (AMSN) supports and conducts research related to medical-surgical nursing practice. The research priorities of AMSN are focused on the current strategic plan. These priorities are listed in order of importance: 1) support, through a funding mechanism, evidence-based practice projects that address clinical practice challenges faced in medical-surgical nursing practice; 2) investigate the effect of certification on the practice of medical-surgical nurses, patient outcomes, and organizations that employ medical-surgical nurses; 3) examine the changing and diverse needs of medical-surgical nurses and awareness of the nursing specialty; 4) investigate the medical-surgical nurse's influence on the selection of clinical products and materials to promote quality patient care, and determine ways to increase this influence; and 5) determine and examine other research priorities that the AMSN membership deems important.

Sue Stott
Academy of Medical-Surgical Nurses
Pitman, NJ

Index

Page numbers appended with *f* or *t* refer to content in figures or tables, respectively.